THE SPANISH FLU PANDEMIC

The Deadliest Pandemic in History and How it Changed the World

by
ELLIOT FRANK

ELLIOT FRANK

Copyright © 2020

All rights reserved. No part of this publication may be reproduced, distributed, or transmitted in any form or by any means, including photocopying, recording, or other electronic or mechanical methods, without the prior written permission of the publisher, except in the case of brief quotations embodied in critical reviews and certain other noncommercial uses permitted by copyright law

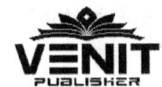

TABLE OF CONTENTS

INTRODUCTION 6

THE ORIGIN 12
   HISTORICAL BACKGROUND 17

PATHOGENESIS OF THE SPANISH FLU 24

GENETIC CHARACTERIZATION 30
   FUTURE WORK 32

ANIMAL ORIGIN 36

WHAT IS THE FLU? 46
   FLU SEASON 46
   WHAT CAUSED THE SPANISH FLU? 47
   WHY WAS IT CALLED THE SPANISH FLU? 49

SYMPTOMS 54
   FLU COMPLICATIONS 55

MORTALITY 58
   CHILD MORTALITY 60
   INACCURATE MORTALITY DATA 63

WHY WAS THE FLU SO DEADLY? 72
   LACK OF QUARANTINE 80
   MEDICAL SCIENCE DID NOT HAVE THE TOOLS 81

MORBIDITY AND SOCIOECONOMICAL INDICES 84
   MATERIALS AND METHODS 87
   RESULTS 90
   DISCUSSION 92

THE FIRST WAVE	**98**
THE SECOND WAVE	**102**
Timeline of The Second Wave	108
THE THIRD WAVE	**112**
HOW DID IT END?	**114**
LACK OF SOCIAL ESTRANGEMENT	**116**
THE 1920'S-1950'S	**120**
POST-TRAUMATIC COMPLICATIONS	**128**
THE ECONOMIC EFFECTS	**138**
Summary of economic research	140
Overview	143
THE SOCIAL IMPACT IN AFRICA	**146**
COULD A 1918 PANDEMIC REAPPEAR?	**150**
PREPARING FOR THE NEXT PANDEMIC	**156**
IMPACT ON MENTAL HEALTH	**160**
Psychological Disorders in Survivors	161
Mourning	165
Care of Mental Health	170
Psychological and Social Care	172
Lines of action	179
ORGANIZATION OF SERVICES.	**182**
DEAD BODY MANAGEMENET	**184**
MASS COMMUNICATION STRATEGIES	**196**
CONCLUSIONS	**202**

ELLIOT FRANK

INTRODUCTION

The Spanish Flu pandemic was one of the deadliest pandemics of the modern era, described as "the greatest medical holocaust in history". Despite the seriousness, it is fair to say that the 1918 Influenza has been almost forgotten as a tragic event in history. This has negative aspects, because learning from the past may be the only way to be reasonably prepared for future pandemics.

The number of deaths caused worldwide is estimated at 40 and 100 million. Other researchers have suggested even higher numbers, which seem somewhat outrageous. However, the emergence and development of the Spanish Flu continues to raise a number of unanswered questions, which must be addressed in light of new flu pandemics.

Our main concern here is to establish where, when and under what circumstances the pandemic began.

Did it start in the spring-summer of 1918, or were there earlier episodes related to the great pandemic?

Does it have any similarity to current pandemics?

We explored reports from medics who served on the lines and assisted the French and American armies during World War I. These documents are kept in the archives of the French army health services in Val-de-Groce (Paris) and military archives in the United States and England. Other sources include medical articles and books published during that period.

Several archives in Africa, Spain and Portugal were also consulted to provide complete information.

As an important background we were able to find that the 1889-1890 pandemic was particularly interesting because of the similarities with the later Spanish Flu. It forms a link between epidemics and pandemics that have occurred in modern times and especially with the extremely virulent Influenza of 1918. Doctors of the time attributed these outbreaks to the remnants of the 1889-1890 pandemic; they considered the Influenza to be an endemic disease. At that time, there was no distinction between seasonal and pandemic influenza, the primary virus having not yet been discovered.

The 1889-1890 pandemic may have occurred in the following countries, among others: China (after the 1888 flood); Athabasca in Canada (May 1889); Greenland (summer 1889), Tomsk in Siberia or Bukhara in Uzbekistan (October 1889). We know for certain that the first cases arose in St. Petersburg (Russia) on October 27,

1889, and quickly spread by rail to all of Europe. In Paris, the first cases were recorded on 17 November, in Berlin and Vienna on 30 November, in London in mid-December and in the countries of southern Europe, from Italy to Portugal in late December. The Influenza spread to the United States in January 1890, with the first cases in Boston and New York. During the first months of the year, it spread to the Americas, Africa, Asia and Oceania, reaching remote islands such as Madagascar, Jamaica and St. Helena in August.

Influenza pandemics, which are distinguished from epidemics by their geographical distribution, have caused significant illness, death and chaos for centuries. However, in recent decades, globalization has led to social and economic changes that have increased the chances of developing a disease and accelerated the spread of new viruses.

In a positive way, globalization has also facilitated international cooperation and promoted progress in disease research and surveillance. Collectively, these processes change the way pandemics emerge, are experienced, understood and controlled.

This book explores how changes in human demographics, economic systems, medical capabilities, and epidemiological practices affected the consequences of the Spanish Flu Pandemic and the approaches and challenges they had to face in responding to outbreaks.

Over the past century, different strains of influenza have emerged, each leading to a global pandemic. These diseases were addressed in turn, highlighting the origin, the reactions and the burden of consequences. This assessment is complemented by an analysis of how changes in the intervening years between plagues, related to the processes of globalization and infectious disease practices, have affected exposure and preparedness for the next pandemic.

From 1918 to the present, in all regions of the inhabited planet we have suffered at least one deadly flu epidemic, with more or less alarming rates, after that catastrophic year, humanity changed the way it reacted to a viral disease, although the officials were not prepared for what happened, considering that the governmental and economic attention was all concentrated on the armament efforts of the time, we can find documentation that allows us to observe the passage and devastation of the Spanish Flu from the hand to the "Great War".

THE ORIGIN

The predominant natural reservoir for influenza viruses is believed to be wild waterfowl. Periodically, genetic material from virus strains is transferred to virus strains that are infectious to humans through a process called rearrangement. Strains of the newly acquired human influenza virus and internal RNA segments encoding proteins were responsible for pandemic influenza outbreaks in 1957 and 1968. The change in the hemagglutinin subtype or the hemagglutinin and neuraminidase subtype is called an antigenic shift. Since pigs can become infected with avian and human virus, they have been proposed as intermediaries in this process. Until recently, there was only limited evidence that a complete avian influenza virus could directly infect humans. In 1997, eighteen people were infected with the H5N1 avian influenza virus in Hong Kong, six died of complications after the infection. Although these viruses were poorly communicable or non-communicable, their isolation from infected patients indicates that humans can become infected with complete strains of avian influenza viruses. H5N1 outbreaks in poultry were widespread in Asia in 2003-2004, at least 23 people died from complications of the infection in Vietnam and Thailand (WHO 2004).

In 2003 an outbreak of highly pathogenic H7N7 occurred on poultry farms in the Netherlands. This virus caused infections (mainly conjunctivitis) in 86 poultry processors and three secondary contacts, one of the infected people died of pneumonia. In 2004, an outbreak of H7N3 influenza in poultry in Canada also caused infection in a single individual (WHO 2004). A patient in New York is said to be ill after infection with an H7N2 virus, therefore, it may not be necessary to involve pigs as intermediaries in the formation of a pandemic virus strain, since reorganization between a bird and a human influenza virus can occur directly in humans. While rearrangement with genes encoding surface, proteins appear to be a critical event for the production of a pandemic virus. There is a large body of data to suggest that influenza viruses also need specific adaptations to spread and replicate efficiently. A new host, among other features should be the functional binding of the HA receptor (Hemagglutinin "HA"" is an antigenic glycoprotein found on the surface of the flu virus) "and the interaction between viral and host proteins. Defining the minimal adaptive changes necessary for a rearranged virus to function in humans is essential to understanding how pandemic viruses originate. Once a new virus strain has undergone the changes that allow it to spread in humans, virulence is affected by the presence of new surface proteins that enable the virus to infect an immunologically naive population. This was the case in 1957 and 1968, and almost certainly was the case in 1918. While immunological novelty may account for much of the virulence of the 1918 influenza, additional genetic traits are likely to have contributed to its exceptional lethality.

Unfortunately, not enough is known about how the genetic characteristics of influenza viruses affect virulence. The degree of disease caused by a particular virus strain or virulence is complicated, it includes host factors such as immune status and viral factors such as host adaptation, transmissibility, tissue tropism, or the efficiency of viral replication. The hereditary reason for every one of these characteristics has not yet been completely portrayed, however, it is almost sure to be polygenic. Before testing for the 1918 virus described in this review, only two pandemic influenza virus strains were available for molecular analysis: the 1957 H2N2 virus strain and the 1968 H3N2 virus strain. The 1957 pandemic resulted in the appearance of a rearrangement. Influenza viruses where HA (Hemagglutinin) and NA (Neuraminidase) were replaced by genetic segments closely related to those of avian virus strains. The 1968 pandemic followed the appearance of a virus strain in which the HA gene of the H2 subtype was exchanged with a segment of H3 RNA derived from birds, while the N2 gene-derived in 1957 was retained. More recently, the PB1 gene has been shown to replace both the 1957 and 1968 pandemic virus strains, also with a possible bird shunt in both cases. The remaining five RNA segments encoding the PA, PB2, nucleoprotein, matrix, and nonstructural proteins were retained from the H1N1 virus strains circulating before 1957.

These segments were likely the direct descendants of the genes present in the 1918 virus. Since only the 1957 and 1968 pandemic influenza virus strains are available for sequence analysis, it is unclear what changes are necessary to strain the virus's occurrence with pandemic potential. Sequence analysis of the 1918 influenza virus allows us to potentially address the genetic basis of virulence and adaptation to humans.

Historical Background

The 1918 influenza pandemic was exceptional in both breadth and depth. Outbreaks of the disease not only flooded North America and Europe but also spread to the Alaskan wilderness and the most remote Pacific islands. It is estimated that one-third of the world population (500 million people) may be clinically infected during the pandemic.

The disease was also exceptionally severe, with death rates among infected people above 2.5 percent, compared to less than 0.1 percent in other influenza epidemics. The total mortality attributable to the 1918 pandemic is likely to be approximately 40 million.

Unlike most subsequent strains of the influenza virus that developed in Asia, the "first wave" or "spring wave" of the 1918 pandemic emerged in the United States in March 1918, however, the almost simultaneous occurrence of influenza in March-April 1918 in North America, Europe, and Asia makes it difficult to finally assign a point of geographic origin. It is possible that a mutation or rearrangement occurred in the late summer of 1918, resulting in significantly improved virulence. The primary wave of the global pandemic, the "fall wave" or "second wave," occurred in September-November 1918, in many places, there was another major Flu wave in early.

Three extensive influenza outbreaks within a year are rare, they may indicate unique features of the 1918 virus that can be revealed in order. Outbreaks of inter-pandemic influenza generally occur in a single annual wave in late winter. The severity of annual outbreaks is affected by antigenic drift, with an antigen-modified virus strain emerging every two to three years, even with pandemic influenza, although regular seasonal influences can be violated in late winter, the succession of clear waves within a year is rare.

The 1890 pandemic began in the late spring of 1889, it lasted for several months and spread throughout the world, peaking in northern Europe and the United States in late 1889 or early 1890, the second wave arose in 1891 (more than a year after the first wave) and the third wave in early 1892 (Jordan 1927). As in 1918, successive waves seemed to cause more severe illness, so maximum mortality was reached in the third wave of the pandemic, however, the three waves spanned over three years, compared to less than a year in 1918. It is unclear what gave the 1918 virus this unusual ability to generate repeated waves of disease, perhaps the virus's surface proteins moved faster than other strains of the influenza virus, or maybe the virus had an unusually effective mechanism for evading the human immune system. Most people who died during the pandemic succumbed to secondary bacterial pneumonia, as antibiotics were not available in 1918, however, a subgroup died soon after the onset of symptoms, often with massive acute pulmonary hemorrhage or pulmonary edema, usually in less than five days. In the hundreds of autopsies performed in 1918, the primary pathologic findings were limited to the respiratory system, and death was due to pneumonia and respiratory failure, these findings are consistent with infection with a well-adapted influenza virus that allows rapid replication throughout the respiratory system, there was no clinical or pathological evidence of systemic virus circulation. Furthermore, in the 1918 pandemic, most deaths occurred among young adults, a group with a very low influenza mortality rate. Influenza and pneumonia death rates in people ages 15 to 34 were more than 20 times higher in 1918 than in previous years. The 1918 pandemic is also unique among Flu pandemics, as the absolute risk of Flu mortality was higher in people younger than 65 than in people older than 65.

Notably, people under the age of 65 were responsible for more than 99 percent of all Flu-related deaths in 1918-1919. In contrast, the age group younger than 65 was responsible for only 36 percent of all influenza-related excess deaths in the 1957 H2N2 pandemic and 48 percent in the 1968 H3N2 pandemic. Overall, nearly half of the influenza-related deaths in the influenza pandemic of 1918 were young adults ages 20 to 40. As another unique feature, had the simultaneous infection of humans and pigs. Interestingly, swine Flu was first recognized as such a clinical entity in the fall of 1918, simultaneously with the spread of the second wave of the pandemic in humans, the researchers were impressed by the clinical and pathological similarities of influenza in humans and pigs in 1918. A full description by veterinarian W. W. Dimock of swine diseases, published in August 1918, does not mention swine Flu-like illness. For example, contemporary researchers were convinced that the influenza virus had not circulated as an epizootic disease in pigs before 1918 and that the virus had spread from man to pig due to the onset of the disease in pigs after the first wave of human Flu of 1918. After that, the disease became widespread among herds of pigs in the Midwestern United States, the epizootic from 1919-20 was as high as in 1918-19. The disease appeared every year among pigs in the Midwest, this led to isolation in 1930, three years before the isolation of the first human influenza virus. Classical swine viruses circulate not only in pigs in North America but also in pig populations in Europe and Asia.

PATHOGENESIS OF THE SPANISH FLU

The Spanish Flu was caused by the H1N1 virus with genes of avian origin. Although there is no general consensus as to where it occurred, it spread worldwide during 1918-1919. Mortality rates were highest among people under 5 and between 20 and 40. The high mortality rate in healthy people, including the 20-40 age group, was a unique feature of this pandemic. Although the 1918 H1N1 virus has been synthesized and evaluated, the characteristics that made it so catastrophic are not clearly determined. With no vaccines to guard against influenza infection and no antibiotics to treat secondary bacterial infections that became associated with influenza infections, worldwide control efforts were restricted to non-pharmacological mediations, such as lockdown, quarantine, good personal hygiene habits, use of antiseptics, and limitations on public meetings, which were carried out unevenly.

Spanish influenza did not originate in Spain. Even so, it is likely that in Europe the deadly virus developed in "Etaples", a huge military camp in northern France. At one point, no less than 100,000 men were found near both pigs and poultry.

In the United States it was first discovered during the spring of 1918, among military personnel while soldiers were waiting to be sent to war in Europe. Starting at Funston Camp in Kansas, the virus spread to other camps and through troop raids to Europe. Within three months, 43,000 US soldiers would have succumbed to the disease. The devastation was hidden by wartime censorship. It was an element of war propaganda that located the origin of the disease in Spain and not in the United States.

The following extract described by doctor Tillson Harrinson provides a brief graphic description of the disease:

"Most flu strains do not kill people directly; instead, death is caused by bacteria flowing into the victim's lungs. But the Spanish flu that circulated in 1918-19 was a direct killer. Victims suffered acute cyanosis, blue discoloration of the skin and mucous membranes, vomiting and coughing up blood, which also flowed uncontrollably from their nose and, in the case of women, from their genitals.

There were a large number of deaths in pregnant women: up to 41 percent of those infected died. If the woman survived, the fetus suffered severe physical and psychological trauma caused by the mother's stress. Many newborns had encephalitis because the virus affected their brain and spinal cord.

Millions of people suffered from acute respiratory distress syndrome, an immune condition in which disease-fighting cells overwhelm the lungs in their fight against invaders and suffocate victims".

On the battlefields of Europe, both enemy and ally, sometimes more than a kilometer away, were infected with the disease. In the trenches and shelters of a terrible war, the disease spread like wildfire and spread the germ for later outbreaks. In the camps for prisoners of war and in the medical transports loaded with wounded veterans, it was impelled even more that the disease spread. By 1919, it can be said that the entire peopled territory of the earth, from the coldest regions to the tropics of sun and heat, was contaminated with the deadly disease. Ultimately, it is estimated that one third of the world's total population suffered from influenza in 1918-1919.

The disease brought the U.S. military and government to their knees. It wasn't until 1933 that a British research team finally isolated and identified the flu virus. In 2005, scientists at the Armed Forces Institute of Pathology in Washington collected samples of the H1N1 virus that started the Spanish flu pandemic and demonstrated its lethality in mice. A year later, a team from Seattle University School of Medicine showed that:

"Mice infected with the reconstructed 1918 flu virus showed an accelerated activation of host immune response genes associated with severe lung disease. They found that mice infected with a virus containing all eight genes of the pandemic virus showed marked activation of pro-inflammatory pathways and consequently in some caused cell death within 24 hours of infection. The virus killed the remaining infected mice within five days, causing their immune systems to go into a frenzy. But, the group of scientists noted that these initial characterizations of the 1918 virus did not address the problem of its pathogenic potential in primates.

Concerned with answering this question, seven healthy macaques were infected. Two animals died from the virus between days three and six, while the remaining animals, originally scheduled for euthanasia on day 21 after infection, died on day 8 because of severe symptoms. In any case, the Spanish Flu, induced in a laboratory or by a natural pathogen, would today be deadly and terrifying in its effect.

GENETIC CHARACTERIZATION

The frozen and fixed lung tissue of five victims of the 1918 fall wave Flu has been used to directly investigate the genetic makeup of the 1918 Flu virus. Two of the cases analyzed were US Army soldiers. They died in September 1918, one at Camp Upton, New York, and the other at Fort Jackson, South Carolina. The available material consists of formalin-fixed and paraffin-embedded autopsy tissue, microscopic sections stained with hematoxylin and eosin, and the medical history of these patients.

Analysis of the crystal structure of HA from 1918 suggests that the overall structure of the receptor-binding site is comparable to that of an H5 HA bird in terms of having a pocket narrower than that identified for human H3 HA. This provides an additional clue to the deviation of birds from HA from 1918, the four antigenic sites identified for another H1 HA, the A / PR / 8/34 HA virus, also appear to be the main antigenic determinants in HA from 1918. X-ray analysis suggests that these sites are exposed in the HA of 1918, which can easily be recognized by the human immune system.

The second mutation with a significant effect on virulence due to pantropism has been identified in the NA gene of two strains of influenza viruses adapted to the mouse, A / WSN / 33, and A / NWS / 33. Mutations appear in a single codon, like the HA cleavage site mutation to allow the virus to replicate in many tissues outside the airways. This mutation was also not observed in the NA of the 1918 virus.

Therefore, none of the genes encoding the surface proteins have known mutations that could make the 1918 virus panoptic. Since the clinical and pathological findings in 1918 showed no evidence of replication outside the respiratory system, it was not expected that the mutations allowed the 1918 virus to replicate systemically, however, the relationship between other structural characteristics of these proteins (apart from their supposed antigenic novelty) and virulence remains unknown. In their general structural and functional characteristics, HA and NA from 1918 are like that of birds, yet they also have characteristics adapted to mammals.

Future Work

The eight 1918 segments of the influenza virus RNA were sequenced and analyzed, their characterization has shed light on the origin of the virus and strongly supports the hypothesis that the 1918 virus was the common ancestor of later human and porcine H1N1 lines. Gene sequence analysis to date does not provide a definitive indication of the genotypic basis for the exceptional virulence of the 1918 virus strain for example, experiments have begun to test virulence models using reverse genetics gene approaches of 1918 influenza.

It is hoped that, in the future, the 1918 pandemic virus strain may be placed in the influenza virus strains that preceded and followed them. The immediate precursor to the pandemic virus, the first strain of the 'spring' wave virus, lacked the exceptional virulence of the last wave virus strain. Identifying a positive RNA case of first wave influenza would be of enormous value in deciphering the genetic basis of virulence, since differences in sequence can be emphasized, identification of human influenza RNA samples before 1918 would clarify which gene segments were new to the virus.

In many ways, the 1918 influenza pandemic was similar to other pandemics, in epidemiology, course of disease, and pathology, in addition, laboratory experiments with recombinant influenza viruses containing genes from the 1918 virus suggest that similar viruses would be as sensitive to FDA-approved Flu rimantadine and oseltamivir medications as other virus strains, however, there are some characteristics of the pandemic that appear to be unique. Mortality was exceptionally high, ranging from five to twenty times greater than usual, clinically and pathologically, the high density of deaths appears to be the result of an increased number of serious and complicated respiratory infections, not a systemic infection or the involvement of organ systems outside the usual targets of the influenza virus. Mortality was concentrated in an unusually young age group that over time, the waves of complaint activity followed surprisingly fast, resulting in three major outbreaks in one year. Each of these unique traits can be explained by the genetic characteristics of the 1918 virus, the challenge will be to determine the links between the biological capabilities of the virus and the known history of the pandemic.

ANIMAL ORIGIN

Viral sequence data now suggest that the entire 1918 virus was new to humans, we did not have a reorganized antibody produced from existing old strains that acquired one or more new genes like those found in the 1957 and 1968 pandemics. By contrast, the 1918 virus appears to be an avian influenza virus that originates from an unknown source, since the eight genome segments are fundamentally different from current avian influenza genes.

The genetic sequences of the influenza virus from several solid samples of wild birds collected around 1918 show little difference from the viruses of currently isolated birds, indicating that bird viruses are likely to undergo small antigenic changes in their natural hosts, even for long periods. For example, the sequence of the 1918 nucleoprotein (NP) gene is similar to that of viruses found in wild birds at the amino acid level, but very diverse at the nucleotide level, suggesting a significant evolutionary distance between sources of NP from 1918 and the currently sequenced NP gene sequence in wild bird species.

One way to see the evolutionary distance of genes is to compare the proportions of synonymous to non-synonymous nucleotide substitutions. Synonymous replacement means silent change, and a nucleotide transforms into a codon that does not result in an amino acid replacement. A non-synonymous substitution is a nucleotide change in a codon that results in an amino acid replacement.

In general, a viral gene that is subject to immunological drift pressure or adapts to a new host exhibits a higher percentage of non-synonymous mutations. In contrast, a virus under low selective pressure mainly accumulates synonymous changes. Since little or no selection pressure is exerted on the synonymous changes, they are believed to reflect evolutionary distance. Given that the 1918 genetic segments show more changes that are synonymous with the sequences of known wild bird species than expected, it is unlikely that they arose directly from an avian influenza virus similar to those sequenced so far.

This is especially evident when examining differences in 4-degenerate codons, the subset of synonymous changes in which, at the third codon position, any of the four possible nucleotides can be replaced without changing the resulting amino acid. Simultaneously, the 1918 sequences have very few amino acid differences from wild bird species to have adapted for years to an intermediate human or porcine host alone. One possible explanation is that these unusual genetic segments were obtained from a reservoir of influenza viruses that have not yet been identified or sampled.

All of these findings raise the question: where does the 1918 virus come from? In contrast to the genetic makeup of the 1918 pandemic virus, the new genetic segments of the reassigned pandemic viruses from 1957 and 1968 all stem from Eurasian avian viruses; both human viruses originated from the same mechanism: rearrangement of a species of wild Eurasian waterfowl with the previously circulating human H1N1 strain.

Testing the hypothesis that the virus responsible for the 1918 pandemic had a distinctly different origin requires samples of human influenza strains circulated before 1918 and samples of influenza strains in nature that are more similar to the 1918 sequences.

What was the biological basis for the pathogenicity of the 1918 pandemic virus? Sequence analysis alone does not indicate the pathogenicity of the 1918 virus. A series of experiments are performed to model virulence in vitro and in animal models using viral constructs containing 1918 genes produced by reverse genetics. The influenza virus infection requires the binding of the HA protein to sialic acid receptors on the host cell's surface.

The configuration of the HA receptor-binding site is different for those influenza viruses adapted to infect birds and those adapted to infect humans. Bird-adapted influenza virus strains bind preferentially to sialic acid receptors with sugars coupled (2-3). Influenza viruses adapted to humans are believed to preferentially bind to α-linked receptors (2-6).

Changing this bird receptor configuration requires the virus to have only one amino acid change, and the HAs of the five sequenced viruses from 1918 has this change, suggesting that it could be a critical step in human host adaptation. A second change may also occur that greatly improves virus binding to the human receptor, but only 3 out of 5 HA sequences of the 1918 virus have it.

This means that at least 2 H1N1 receptor-binding variants circulated in 1918: 1 with high-affinity binding to the human receptor and 1 with mixed affinity binding to both avian and human receptors. There are no geographical or chronological indications to suggest that one of these variants was the precursor to the other, nor are there consistent differences between the clinical cases or the histopathological characteristics of the patients infected with them.

It is unknown whether the viruses were equally transmissible in 1918, whether they had identical replication patterns in the respiratory tree, whether one or both circulated in the first and third pandemic waves.

Recombinant influenza viruses containing between 1 and 5 genetic segments of the 1918 virus have been produced in a series of "in vivo" experiments. Those constructs bearing the 1918 HA (Hemagglutinin) and NA (Neuraminidase) are all highly pathogenic in mice. In addition, expression microarray analysis (is a developing technology to study the expression of many genes at once) performed on whole lung tissue from mice infected with the 1918 recombinant HA / NA showed increased upregulation of genes involved in apoptosis, tissue damage, and oxidative damage. These findings are unexpected because viruses with the 1918 genes did not adapt to mice; Control experiments in which mice were infected with modern human viruses showed little disease and limited viral replication.

The lungs of animals infected with the 1918 HA/NA construct showed bronchial and alveolar epithelial necrosis, and a clear inflammatory infiltrate, suggesting that it contains 1918 HA (and possibly NA) virulence factors for mice. The viral genotypic basis for this pathogenicity has not yet been mapped. It is not clear whether pathogenicity in mice effectively models pathogenicity in humans.

The potential role of the other 1918 proteins, individually and in combination, is also unknown. Experiments are planned to further map the genetic basis for the virulence of the 1918 virus in various animal models. These experiments may help define the viral component of the unusual pathogenicity of the 1918 virus, but cannot determine whether host-specific factors were responsible for unique patterns of influenza mortality in 1918.

ELLIOT FRANK

WHAT IS THE FLU?

The Flu or influenza is a virus that affects the airways. The Flu virus is highly contagious: when an infected person coughs, sneezes or speaks, airborne droplets are generated that can then be inhaled by anyone nearby, also, a person who touches something with the virus and then touches their mouth, eyes, or nose can become infected. Flu outbreaks occur every year and vary in severity, depending in part on what type of virus is being spread.

Flu season

In the United States, the "Flu season" generally runs from late fall through spring. In a typical year, more than 200,000 Americans are hospitalized for Flu-related complications. In the past three decades, there have been between 3,000 and 49,000 Flu-related deaths in the United States each year, according to the Centers for Disease Control and Prevention.

Young children, those over 65, pregnant women, and people with certain medical conditions, such as asthma, diabetes, or heart disease, are at increased risk for Flu-related complications, such as pneumonia, ear infections, and sinusitis, and bronchitis. A Flu pandemic, like the one in 1918, occurs when a particularly virulent new strain of Flu with little or no immunity spreads rapidly from person to person throughout the world.

What caused the Spanish Flu?

The outbreak began in 1918, during the closing months of World War I, and historians now believe that the conflict may have been in part responsible for the spread of the virus. On the western front, soldiers who lived in tight, dirty and wet conditions were easily ill, this was the direct result of a weakened immune system due to malnutrition, many diseases, especially the flu, were contagious and spread between the ranks, about three days after getting sick, many soldiers would start to feel better, but not all of them would. In the summer of 1918, when the troops began to return home on leave, they inadvertently brought the virus that had made them sick. The virus spread to cities and towns on the soldiers' lands, many of the infected, both soldiers and civilians, did not recover quickly. The virus was pronounced in young adults between the ages of 20 and 30 who had previously been healthy.

In 2014, a new theory about the origin of the virus suggested that it first appeared in China, National Geographic reported. Previously undiscovered records linked the Flu to the transportation of Chinese workers, the Chinese Corps of Labor, across Canada in 1917 and 1918, according to Mark Humphries' book "The Last

Plague", they spent six days in sealed train containers as they transported them across the country before heading to France. They had to dig trenches, unload trains, build tracks, build roads, and repair damaged tanks. In total, more than 90,000 workers were mobilized to the Western Front. Humphries explains that in a count of 25,000 Chinese workers, in 1918, about 3,000 completed their Canadian trip. Due to racist stereotypes, his illness was attributed to "Chinese laziness" and Canadian doctors did not take workers' symptoms seriously. When workers arrived in northern France in early 1918, many were ill, and hundreds soon died.

Why was it called the Spanish Flu?

Spain was one of the first countries to detect the epidemic, yet historians believe it was likely due to wartime censorship.

Spain was a neutral country during the war, did not maintain strict censorship of its press, which was therefore free to publish the first reports of the disease, people mistakenly believed that the disease was specific to that country, and the Name "Spanish Flu" was rooted in popular speaking. Even in the late spring of 1918, a Spanish news service sent a message to the Reuters London office, it informed the news agency that "a strange epidemic has developed in Madrid. The epidemic is mild, and there are no deaths reported". Two weeks after the report, more than 100,000 people had been infected with the Flu. The disease hit the king of Spain, Alfonso XIII, along with prominent politicians. Between 30% and 40% of people who worked or lived in confined spaces, such as schools, barracks, and government buildings, were infected. Service on the Madrid tram system had to be reduced, and the telegraph service was discontinued because there were not enough health workers to work. Medical supplies and services were unable to meet demand. The term "Spanish Flu" was quickly adopted in Britain. According to Niall Johnson's book "Great Britain and the Flu Pandemic 1918-19", the British press attributed the blame for the epidemic to Spain: "the dry and windy Spanish spring is an unpleasant and unhealthy season". It was suggested that the microbial-laden dust was spread by strong winds in Spain and they believed that Britain's humid climate could halt the spread of the Flu. In short, the "Spanish Flu" is what the 1918 pandemic Flu is called because many people heard for the first time that it was from Spain, so they thought that this was also the source of the Flu, however, it probably started in elsewhere, but due to World War I, the news only came to light after the cases were reported in Spanish newspapers that they were still working

The global magnitude and spread of the pandemic were exacerbated by the war, which estimated that some 10 million civilians and 9 million soldiers died. The massive movement of troops around the world spreads the disease, tens of thousands of troops died as a result of the Flu pandemic instead of fighting.

Although deaths from the battles of World War I have increased death rates in participating countries, civilian deaths from the 1918 Flu pandemic tended to be much higher. For the United States, estimates of combat-related troop deaths are approximately one-tenth of civilian deaths from the 1918 Flu pandemic. Death rates from the typical Flu are generally higher for very young and very old people, what made the 1918 Flu unique, was that death rates were higher for the 20- to 40-year-old segment of the population, and even more so for men than for women in this age group. Overall, death was not caused by the influenza virus itself, but by the body's immune response to the virus. People with the strongest immune system died more frequently than people with the weakest immune system. A source reports that of the 272,500 male influenza deaths in 1918, nearly 49 percent were between the ages of 20 and 39, while only 18 percent were under the age of 5, and 13 percent were over the age of 50. The fact that men between 18 and 40 years old were the most affected by the Flu had serious economic consequences for families who lost their primary breadwinner. As discussed later in the report, the significant loss of workforces of the highest working-age also had economic consequences for companies.

SYMPTOMS

The symptoms of the "Spanish Flu" were very similar to the symptoms of all the influenza virus strains. It would start with symptoms of the upper respiratory tract, such as the runny nose and stuffy, cough, and sneezing. After that, muscle and joint pain and fever generally began, with fever often very high, in the range of 104 degrees F, and marked by fatigue. Sometimes that was the extent of the symptoms, which ended in a week. But for many, respiratory symptoms would progress to pneumonia, and the body would increase defenses, often to the point of a "cytokine storm," which was generally fatal. A cytokine storm is believed to have been the cause of many, if not most, of the 1918 pandemic deaths. It is an overreaction of the immune system; a respiratory infection causes the body to release massive amounts of Fluid to Flush out the infection and immune cells, these Fluids and cells travel to the lungs so fast that they can accumulate and close the airways. Respiratory failure and death can occur, especially in young, healthy infected individuals with a robust immune system that could produce excessively strong reactions.

Flu complications

Most people who get the Flu will recover in a few days to less than two weeks. Some will develop complications (such as pneumonia) from the Flu, some of which can be life-threatening and lead to death. Sinus and ear infections are examples of moderate complications from the Flu. At the same time, pneumonia is a severe complication can be the result of infection with the influenza virus, a coinfection of the virus or the flu bacteria. Other possible serious complications caused by the Flu include inflammation of the heart (myocarditis), brain (encephalitis) or muscle tissue (myositis, rhabdomyolysis), and multi-organ failure (e.g., respiratory and kidney failure). Infection can cause an extreme inflammatory reaction in the body and lead to sepsis, the body's life-threatening response to infection, can also worsen chronic medical problems, for example, people with asthma may have attacks and people with heart disease may experience a worsening of this condition due to the Flu. Anyone can get sick from the Flu (even healthy people), and serious Flu-related problems can occur, still, some people are at high risk of developing serious Flu-related complications if they get sick. This includes people over the age of 65, people of any age with certain chronic medical conditions (such as asthma, diabetes, or heart disease), pregnant women, and children under the age of 5, but especially those under the age of 2.

MORTALITY

Towards the end of World War I, the world was affected by the influenza pandemic ravages. The disease spread rapidly across the world with an alarming lack of discrimination as to who attacked it and a tendency to pneumonic complications, leading to a massive relative increase in mortality in young adults. In the 1920s, it was estimated that between spring 1918 and early summer 1919, the disease affected 200 to 700 million people and killed 10 to 21 million people. In 1991, David Patterson and Gerald Pyle raised the estimates to between 24.7 million and 39.3 deaths, still, Ian Mills discovered a death toll of more than 21 million in India alone.

The latest reviews have raised the likely global mortality for influenza to between 40 and 100 million, even conservative estimates estimate that the death toll from Flu is more than double that of the World War I, but while the war took responsibility for creating a "lost generation," the "Flu" was quickly relegated to oblivion.

The experience of war and its consequences in terms not only of mortality but also of social and economic reorganization (at least in the United Kingdom, the arrival of the armistice during the most virulent period of the epidemic) must have changed the public perspective and reduced the memory of the pandemic.

While widespread disease undoubtedly imposed additional burdens on society and the economy, these appear primarily included in the experience of war itself. The Flu pandemic investigation, after a mostly inactive period, has recently taken off, this has resulted in better estimates of mortality, morbidity and descriptions of the course of the epidemic and response patterns. These more recent studies focused on disproportionate mortality among adults, which was very alarming for those who experienced it, further depleting the generations most affected by the war and increasing social and economic turmoil.

The completely abnormal vulnerability of those at their best was in stark contrast to the usual age pattern of influenza mortality, which was higher between the younger and older groups.

Child mortality

Using an individual level dataset of 30,488 babies born between January 1917 and December 1922 to view mortality rates, identify infants at highest risk during the epidemic and assess the direct, indirect, and associated effects of the epidemic Flu in the health and survival of infants and children.

Anthony Burgess's experience, reflects an unusual age pattern. Anthony's mother, a healthy young woman, and his four-year-old sister died while he was saved just over a year old.

Although they experienced the largest proportional increases in death rates between the ages of twenty and thirty, usually very low for those age groups under normal conditions. The absolute number of deaths among infants and children under the age of five remained significant.

Christopher Langford has suggested that the unusual pattern of the 1918-1919 pandemic was due to immunity conferred by previous epidemics in the elderly, and that mortality among younger age groups was not abnormally low.

Babies and young children are a particularly vulnerable group in all circumstances, just one year before the pandemic, nearly 10 percent of babies born in England and Wales died before their first birthday.

It was concluded that the impact of World War I on British society was inextricably related to the Flu epidemic, still, because very young children were not as involved in the war as adults (although the possible effects of the war on children's health should not be forgotten), research on infants and children can provide an opportunity to separate the results of the pandemic from those of war. This does not mean that the influenza pandemic effect on infants and young children can be extrapolated to adults; in fact, shows that there can be several mechanisms by which influenza can affect the health of boys and girls.

Inaccurate mortality data

Comparing data from censuses conducted during the pandemic in different countries and throughout the 20th century, we can find a systematic variation in the percentage of deaths within the population infected by the virus, important data were voluntarily hidden so as not to affect the morale of soldiers and others were simply lost as a direct consequence of war, entire countries were excluded from the calculation due to lack of population records or disorganization.

A recent article by Lancet, which unfortunately did not include African data, extrapolates mortality rates from 1918-19 among the world population in 2004. It indicates that approximately 62 million people would be wiped out by a similar influenza pandemic. The authors noted that they had identified all countries with high quality population censuses for the 1918-19 pandemic and used them to calculate excess mortality.

In combination with various census materials, the authors' statistical analysis of the correlation between births and mortality during the 1918 pandemic indicated a linear and logarithmic relationship in which it increased by 10%.

Due to the lack of "high-quality vital registration data" for the African pandemic, the authors have excluded all countries on the African continent from their argument. This is unfortunate, mainly because if the pandemic presented in the article were reconsidered, no less than 29% of the estimated total deaths would occur in sub-Saharan Africa, a region that represented 11.3% of the world's population.

In India, based on his findings, Professor Christopher Murray concluded that, in the 1918 pandemic, "the most decisive factor was that census record material in colonial India substantially influenced the table of estimates of mortality by pandemic, based on key registration evidence clearly indicating the anomaly provided by the data".

The authors indicated that excess mortality ranged from 0.2% in Denmark to 7.8% in the central provinces of India and Berar. The authors even noted that the calculated average mortality rate in the nine Indian areas was 4.4% and could have been even higher. Furthermore, if one could compare the accurate household data in Denmark and the imprecision in rural India, the vast dominance of the nine Indian provinces in the material analyzed suggested that the findings could be significantly biased by the Indian data.

Due to the lack of high-quality registration data, Murray and colleagues deliberately chose to exclude Africa. However, the material available in the Kew National Archives provides us with data that can be used to modify the findings.

To illustrate that there is sufficient archival material available that can be used to supplement the data used by Murray and his colleagues with African data for the 1918 pandemic, the following section (based on material collected from the Kew National Archives) provides a brief description of the course of the pandemic in three of the British colonies in West Africa.

In the wake of the pandemic, efforts have been made to determine the extent to which certain groups of individuals have been affected, although this information was scarce. In a report prepared by the Medical Director of Freetown, it was noted that "it is not easy to determine even approximate numbers of people affected by the disease". To determine the mortality of the epidemic, it was hoped that "since registration is compulsory, more or less accurate figures could be obtained" but it turned out that this was not the case.

At the height of the epidemic, several bodies were buried without a death certificate, and cemetery personnel were so limited by the disease that there is reason to believe that not all funerals were included in the funeral records. Even as the pandemic spread, it is clear that many fled jobs that involved the treatment of infected bodies, leaving the control of population records as a last priority for the authorities.

In Sierra Leone, when investigating the impact of the pandemic, British medical and health officials in Freetown used the 1911 census, which recorded a population of 34,000. The official believed that the number of deaths from influenza since August 23, 1918, when the beginning of the pandemic was recognized in that city and September 18, 1918, when it ended, was 968.

The total deaths are likely to be much higher than the numbers show. It is generally believed that at least one thousand of the civilian population (European and indigenous) in Freetown died from the disease. While the figures for the total population of Freetown may be inaccurate, the military records of the troops and their families stationed in Freetown claim to be accurate and in addition to the Secretary-General's figures. The total population of the garrison, including women and children, was 3,282, of whom 2,368 (71.1 per cent) were diagnosed with influenza. In total, 68 people died, 2.87 per cent of the garrison population.

The police, who had no barracks, came from most of the tribes in Freetown and can be considered among the different classes of natives affected. Living as part of the civilian population, their level of infection and mortality was the same as that of other men of the same age and standard of living in the city. As a police force, this group was accurately recorded and any absence was immediately reported. Of a force of 180, 130 were reported sick and diagnosed with the flu, an incidence of 72.2 percent.

The prison services, by their very nature, like the police and the army, scrupulously monitored all prisoners, and it can be reasonably assumed that their data were correct. Of the 290 prisoners, 256 had "severe flu", while the remaining 34 had a "mild attack", i.e. all the prisoners had the disease, however, being infected together with prison workers, including the nursing staff, they had privileged means and care, at that very historical moment there was no overcrowding so the prisoners were unexpectedly successful. In the words of the official report of the time:

"The prison figures show that, as the cases were noticed in time, thanks to the confinement and consequent distancing from the civilian population, timely treatment was possible, internally they possessed agricultural means for self-support and obtained good nutrition, the prisoners had a considerably lower mortality rate than the ordinary resident who stayed in the city in many cases".

WHY WAS THE FLU SO DEADLY?

The dire extent of the pandemic is difficult to understand, the virus infected 500 million people worldwide, killing some 40 to 100 million, more than all of the soldiers and civilians killed together during World War I, while the global pandemic lasted for two years, a significant number of deaths happened in three particularly brutal months in the fall of 1918. Historians now believe that a mutated virus caused the deadly severity of the "second wave" of the Spanish Flu, troop movements spread rapidly in times of war.

When the Spanish Flu first appeared in early March 1918, it had all the characteristics of the seasonal Flu, however, it was a highly contagious and virulent strain.

One of the first recorded cases was Albert Gitchell, a US Army cook in Camp Funston,

Kansas, hospitalized with a 104-degree fever. The virus spread rapidly through the army facility, home to 54,000 soldiers and by the end of the month, 1,100 soldiers had been hospitalized, and 38 had died of pneumonia.

While American troops were deployed in masse for the war effort in Europe, they carried the Spanish Flu. In April and May 1918, the virus spread like wildfire across England, France, Spain, and Italy. Estimated three-quarters of the French army were infected in the spring of 1918 and as many as half of the British troops, still, the first wave of the virus didn't seem particularly deadly, with symptoms like high fever and general malaise generally lasting only three days. According to limited public health data at the time, death rates were comparable to seasonal Flu.

From September to November 1918, the mortality rate from the Spanish Flu increased enormously. In the United States alone, only 195,000 Americans died in October and unlike a normal seasonal Flu, which mainly affects very young and very old people, the second wave of Spanish Flu showed a so-called "W curve": a high number of deaths among young and old, but also a massive spike in the medium made up of healthy people from 20 to 40 years old.

It was shocking not only that millions of young men and women died worldwide, but also how they died. Battered by searing fever, nosebleeds, and pneumonia, patients drowned in their Fluid-filled lungs. It was only decades later that scientists were able to explain the phenomenon now known as "cytokine explosion."

When a virus attacks the human body, the immune system sends messenger proteins called cytokines to promote beneficial inflammation, but some Flu strains, especially the H1N1 strain responsible for the Spanish Flu outbreak, can cause a dangerous immune response in healthy individuals. In those cases, the body is overloaded with cytokines, causing severe inflammation and deadly Fluid buildup in the lungs. British military doctors who perform autopsies on soldiers killed by the second wave described severe lung damage as similar to the effects of chemical warfare.

Why did the 1918 virus kill so many healthy young adults? The mortality curve for different types of influenza at the age of death has been U-shaped for at least 150 years and shows peaks of mortality in very young and very old people, with a relatively low frequency of deaths at all intermediate ages. In contrast, the age-specific death rates in the 1918 pandemic showed a clear pattern that has not been documented before or after a W-shaped curve, similar to the U-shaped curve but with the addition of a third clear (average) peak of deaths in young adults aged 20 to 40 years.

For example, influenza and pneumonia death rates for those 15–34 years old in 1918–1919 were 20 times higher than in previous years. Overall, nearly half of the Flu-related deaths during the 1918 pandemic were in young adults in their 20s and 40s, a phenomenon unique to that pandemic year. The 1918 pandemic is also unique among influenza pandemics, as the absolute risk of death from influenza was higher in individuals under age 65 than in individuals over 65; people under the age of 65 were responsible for 99% of all flu-related deaths in 1918-1919.

By comparison, the under-65 age group was responsible for 36% of all influenza-related deaths la in the 1957 H2N2 pandemic and 48% in the 1968 H3N2 pandemic. A sharper perspective arises when Age-specific influenza morbidity rates (21) since 1918 have been used to fit the W-shaped mortality curve. Persons under 35 years of age in 1918 had a disproportionately high incidence of influenza.

However, even after adjusting for age-specific clinical attacks, a W-shaped curve with a peak in deaths among young adults remains and differs significantly from cases of specific U-shaped mortality curves, the age typically observed in other influenza years, for example, 1928 –1929. In addition, in 1918, individuals between the ages of 5 and 14 had a disproportionately large percentage of flu cases, but had a much lower mortality rate from influenza and pneumonia than other age groups.

Different risk factors such as co-infections, drugs and the environment, one theory that may partially explain these findings is that the 1918 virus had an intrinsically high virulence, which was only attenuated in patients born before 1889, for example, by exposure to a virus that was circulating at the time and could provide partial immune protection against the 1918 virus only in people who were old enough (over 35) to become infected during that period.

But this theory would provide an additional paradox: an obscure progenitor virus that left no detectable trace should have appeared and disappeared before 1889, and reappeared more than three decades later. Epidemiological data on the extent of clinical influenza by age, collected between 1900 and 1918, provide good evidence for the emergence of a new antigenic influenza virus in 1918.

U.S. Public Health Service door-to-door studies in eight states during 1919 showed a more typical curve for age-specific flu deaths. The 5- to 15-year-old age group increased to 25% of flu cases (consistent with exposure to a new strain of antigenic virus). The 65-year-old age group accounted for only 0.6% of influenza cases, findings consistent with previously acquired protective immunity caused by an identical or closely related viral protein to which the elderly were once exposed. Mortality rates are consistent; in 1918, people aged 20-40 years who had the flu and cases of pneumonia died in higher percentages. At the other end of the age spectrum, a large proportion of deaths in infants and young children in 1918 mimicked the age pattern of other influenza pandemics.

Lack of Quarantine

The rapid spread of the Spanish Flu in the fall of 1918 is believed to have been partly responsible for public health officials who were unwilling to quarantine during the war.. For example, in Britain, a government official named Arthur Newsholme knew very well that strict civil closure was the best way to combat the spread of the highly contagious disease, but he would not risk paralyzing the war effort by keeping munition factory workers and other civilians at home.

According to our research, Newsholme concluded that "the unwavering needs of war justify justifying the risk of spreading the infection" and encouraged the British to just continue during the pandemic.

A severe shortage of nurses further hampered the public health response to the crisis in the

United States. Thousands of nurses had been deployed to military camps and the front line, the deficit was compounded by the American Red Cross's refusal to use trained African American nurses until the worst pandemic had passed.

Medical science did not have the tools

But one of the main reasons that the Spanish Flu claimed so many lives in 1918 was that science simply did not have the means to develop a vaccine against the virus. Until the 1930s, microscopes couldn't even see something as small as a virus, instead, the best medical professionals in 1918 were convinced that the Flu was caused by a bacterium called "Pfeiffer's bacillus".

After a worldwide Flu outbreak in 1890, a German doctor named Richard Pfeiffer discovered that all of his infected patients carried a certain strain of bacteria that he called "H. Influenza". When the pandemic occurred, scientists planned to find a cure for the Pfeiffer bacillus. In December 1918, the deadly second wave of the Spanish Flu finally ended, but the pandemic was far from over. A third wave broke out in Australia in January 1919 and finally returned to Europe and the United States, president Woodrow Wilson is believed to have contracted the Spanish Flu during the World War I peace negotiations in Paris in April 1919. The death rate for the third wave was as high as the second wave, but the end of the war in November 1918 removed the conditions that allowed it to spread as fast and as far. Global third wave deaths, while still in the millions, paled compared to apocalyptic losses during the second wave.

MORBIDITY AND SOCIOECONOMICAL INDICES

Morbidity is the number of people who get sick in a given place and time period relative to the total population. In 20th century literature it was argued that this pandemic infected and killed all classes equally, however, later studies questioned the "socially neutral vision" of the devastation left by the Flu.

They found higher mortality among the poor in several socio-economic rates, including per capita income, municipalities, occupational classes, homes sizes, literacy, housing type, health care and unemployment. Contemporary studies have shown mixed associations between socioeconomic status and morbidity.

First, control age, gender and race using data from 9 US cities. In the fall of 1918, the United States found a negative association between the financial status of an individual (very poor, poor, middle class, and rich) and morbidity.

Second, a study in Bergen, Norway, which analyzed three waves in combination, found a moderately negative relationship between the number of rooms and morbidity.

Third, studies from 5 English cities, which combined data from 3 waves, found no association between people per room and morbidity in 3 of the cities and a positive correlation in 2.

Finally, a Boston study with data from the fall of 1918 found no difference in morbidity for districts (very poor, poor, moderate), but individuals per room and cleanliness (very dirty, dirty, clean, very clean) were positively and negatively associated with morbidity, respectively.

Without data to analyze the relationship between socioeconomic status and morbidity, it was concluded that they had no relation to the death toll. Testing for other locations cannot be used for this analysis because, at that time, the data was only collected for the wave in late 1918.

Recently, an investigation into morbidity and social classes has been required, confronting the cross-data in the different waves of the Spanish Flu, however, it has not been carried out due to the lack of data.

It is essential for several reasons, first, determining whether economic groups have greater morbidity can help with potential or scarce vaccines, reduce human, social and financial losses in an upcoming pandemic.

Second, morbidity studies would help to understand whether a nation's economics and job stability can influence exposure/morbidity, lethality, or both.

Materials and Methods

The data comes from an investigation into the pandemic in Bergen, Norway. Eight districts were randomly selected, this strategy ensured homes with and without Flu cases.

The risk age and mortality distributions for influenza in the sample and the population were the same. Trained nurses interviewed all families from late 1918 to late 1919, and the data was classified and published based on observed waves from July-September 1918, October-December 1918, and January-March 1919. The sample consists of 10,633 individuals, 4,818 cases, and 72 deaths and covers 11.8% of the population.

Individual data has been lost, but outcome data sorted by age, sex and location of residence have been published and used. Data on outcomes and population at risk is also available by age and gender.

The results did not cause serious differences in the mortality rate by age, sex and wave due to the few deaths in the sample, however, particular features have been documented; significantly higher male mortality, W-shaped mortality (increases and decreases relatively) and higher second wave mortality.

The outcome variable is the probability that an influenza-like illness (ILI) could also have been considered during each wave, that is, cases of ILI are part of the percentage of the population at risk at the beginning of the wave considered.

The risk population at the beginning of the autumn and winter waves is adjusted for cases during the summer and autumn waves, respectively, given that 6.5% of the respondents reported reinfection during the autumn and winter waves, only a factor of 0.935 of the cases of summer wave and the autumn wave is subtracted from the population at risk at the beginning of the autumn wave and the winter wave, respectively.

Explanatory variables are on socioeconomic indexes, home, gender and wave. The address is measured in the number of rooms per house.

The apartment categories are as follows (% sample):
- One room with/without a kitchen (31%)
- Two rooms with kitchen (31%)
- Three rooms with kitchen (15%)
- Four or more rooms with kitchen (22%)

The analysis was performed for the three waves.

Results

The results strongly suggest that women living in two-bedroom apartments had higher morbidity (significant at 10%). If we compare the two smallest types of apartments with the two largest and do not take gender into account, morbidity was significantly lower among residents of larger apartments.

The entire pandemic period hides fundamental differences. In the summer, both men and women living in 3- and 4-bedroom apartments had significantly lower mortality rates.

One in 3 and 1 in 5 in the two smallest and two largest apartment categories had the Flu. These differences were significant at the 0.1% level for men and women and the 1% level for both sexes. The results suggest that women living in two-bedroom apartments had a higher percentage.

A transition from morbidity to department size occurred from summer to fall. In the fall, more men and women were gradually infected by apartment size. The trend is clear, and those who live in apartments with more than four rooms, regardless of gender, tend to have the highest morbidity (significant at 10%). In the winter of 1919, morbidity differences by apartment size and male and female gender were negligible.

However, in studies conducted with hospitalized patients with Flu symptoms and who shared a room, they had the highest mortality rate (30-32%), showing that reduced environments, overcrowding and distance, influenced aggressively to the spread of the virus.

Discussion

Overcrowding is related to poverty, but it also directly promotes the spread of infectious diseases. Residents of small apartments are likely to have higher-exposure, working-class occupations than large apartments with upper/middle-class occupations. Preliminary investigations for Norway showed that those who became ill during the summer were transport, hotel, and industrial workers.

A second candidate is a socioeconomic variation among families exposed to the summer wave, in several Norwegian cities, those who were on vacation were not at risk, on the contrary those who stayed in the city were directly exposed. A study of the 1918-1919 pandemic in Oslo found that apartments' size was perfectly correlated with monthly rent and family income.

Household income and rooms are common indicators of the socioeconomic index in health studies, as it is noted that more families live in large houses, the probability that they can afford a summer vacation increases.

Therefore, the chances of higher-income families being exposed to the summer wave and receiving immunity to combat the fall outbreak may have been lower than that of the poorest families. This hypothesis is consistent with the Oslo finding, children from wealthy families on the west side were more absent due to the fall Flu than children from low-income families on the east side.

A third candidate is the hand hygiene. A 1918 Boston study found that a higher proportion of "cleaner" families had no or had only one case of Flu than "dirty" homes. A review of influenza epidemics found that hand hygiene in community institutions affected influenza transmission. Bergen health authorities urged people to wash their hands and houses, this alert information was printed in newspapers and posters in 1918, still, fewer poor people are likely to know the importance of the messages.

In Oslo, there was a strong negative correlation between 1918 influenza mortality and the availability of homes (richer) with bath. Therefore, having a bath is probably associated positively with hand hygiene and negatively with morbidity.

Those who lived in larger apartments in Bergen are more likely to have bathrooms than those in smaller apartments. Therefore, this presumption could also explain why the highest socioeconomics groups in Bergen had a lower contagion rate in the summer of 1918.

Occupation, occupational exposure, separation from summer vacation in higher socioeconomic groups and hand hygiene are possible mechanisms for differential exposure and transmission of influenza, however, people with lower incomes also they may have more vulnerable immune function, derived from food, poor quality medical care, and social pressures, which increased the risk of developing the Flu when exposed. For example, they were more likely to get sick when experimentally exposed to common influenza viruses.

While this analysis was unable to unravel the mechanisms of contagion, the results suggest that preparedness plans should investigate how a pharmaceutical intervention can address differences in morbidity in socioeconomic strata.

Surprisingly, however, social inequalities in the outcomes of the Spanish Flu pandemic are not part of the debate in international preparedness plans for future pandemic Flu.

THE FIRST WAVE

In the United States, unusual influenza activity was first detected in military camps and in some cities during the spring of 1918. The severity and spread of the disease were not reported in the United States and in other countries involved in the war. During the war, the authorities were interested in maintaining high morale among the population and did not want to provide information on diseases that affected soldiers in times of war. Hundreds of thousands of American soldiers crossed the Atlantic to enlist in the war. The massive displacement of troops helped with the spread of influenza worldwide.

These outbreaks that occurred in the spring are now considered the "first wave" of the pandemic; the cases of disease were limited and much milder than those that would be observed during the following two waves.

In Boston the most affected of the civilian population were male workers (47%) followed by housewives (37%), school-age children (11%), out-of-school children (3%). One explanation for the gender difference could be that young adults are more likely to be exposed to the Flu during the first wave of work, whether in the summer or fall. Most of the adult women were housewives, improving protection against the following waves. Summer and fall morbidity were negatively and significantly correlated only for men.

Unlike studies in belligerent countries, where data on young adult males is distorted because many of them were at war, the analyzes for Bergen, the Norwegian city, come from a neutral country that is not war-biased. Data for this city is available for three waves, while those for the United States and the United Kingdom collected data for the fall wave only or published inaccurate data for all waves combined. Two weaknesses of this study are that there is no data available at the individual level, and they were self-reported and not laboratory confirmed. Therefore, some cases could be mistaken for respiratory illnesses other than the Flu. The poor first got the Flu and were generally the most affected. In contrast, the rich with less exposure in the first wave were infected in a higher percentage in the second wave. This finding is in line with previous studies showing that the poor had the highest pandemic mortality in 1918.

THE SECOND WAVE

The second wave of the Spanish Flu was in large percentage, worse than the first. Experts said it was not due to a decline in care, but rather that its harmfulness lay in a probable metamorphosis of the virus, the difficulty of confinement and the need to work in the context of World War I.

The second outbreak, which occurred in September and was the true 1918 influenza pandemic, probably one of the strains of the virus, mutated, became more selective and stimulated mortality, exterminating some 40 million people worldwide. To justify the high mortality of the second wave by the indifference of the population is inappropriate, the main reason was the virus itself, which mutated and became much more deadly.

It is likely that one of the strains of the virus, responsible for the Spanish Flu, was transformed, became more virulent and caused the chaos that engulfed the entire northern hemisphere between September and November 1918.

Certainly, for the people of that time, the Flu was not a serious illness and did not justify the measures we call isolation today. Neither medicine nor the health systems were as developed as we are today, the population did not have effective means of information and they were not informed about what they had to do. Also, the lack of some modern devices such as refrigerators, televisions, cell phones or computers, made isolation a complicated reality and did not convey the need to distance themselves from the way it has been done during modern pandemics.

The conversation about the Spanish Flu pandemic is not exclusive to today. Experts have made similar comparisons between all recent pandemics to better contextualize and understand the crisis they generate. But many of these comparisons do not emphasize the grim realities of the 1918 pandemic. Less sophisticated health care systems and medical technology, the lack of an international world governments organization, and an ongoing world war have helped make it known as the worst pandemic in human history.

The conversation about the Flu pandemic a century ago is not exclusive to social media users. Experts have made similar comparisons between the two pandemics to better contextualize and understand the crisis. But many of these comparisons do not emphasize the grim realities of the 1918 pandemic. Less sophisticated health care systems and medical technology, the lack of an intergovernmental organization of world government, and an ongoing world war have helped make it known as the worst pandemic of human history.

The deadly second wave of the 1918 Spanish flu pandemic may have clues about the current circumstances. This is one of those rare occasions when historians can more or less agree that there are lessons to be learned that are quite simple and can be applied to the present. More than 100 years ago, the Spanish flu was responsible for the deaths of at least 50 million people worldwide: 55,000 in Canada and 675,000 in the United States, many of them between the ages of 20 and 40.

We now have the means to accelerate procedures and think about effective public health policies that can save many lives.

Uncertain data

Investigators have continued to explore the Spanish Flu. The exact number of deaths and the death rate per case, the total number of deaths outside of the total number of registered cases, is unknown due to incomplete and inaccurate data in some less developed regions. In 1918, the registration of death certificates and epidemiology were still premature, many parts of the world were not connected to others, therefore, data cannot be obtained from some of the sources that were precarious at that time.

The statement that the Spanish Flu occurred in several waves is correct, however, the number is still in dispute, these waves began in March 1918 and ended in the summer of 1919.

Most of the deaths in the United States occurred in the fall of 1918, but the exact amount for each wave is unknown. Experts say the second wave was more severe because of the genetic mutation, the wartime movement, and more often associated with bacterial pneumonia, according to a 1991 study. Many experts say that 2.5% is too low and the figures often referred to by many media and academics (2.5% death rate, 500 million people infected and 40 million to 100 million deaths) are contradictory.

If the Spanish flu infected 500 million and killed 40 to 100 million, the number of deaths was 10 to 20 percent. If the death rate was 2.5 percent and if 500 million were infected, the number of deaths was 12.5 million. In 1918 there were 1.8 billion people, combining 40 million deaths with 2.5 percent would require at least 2 billion infections, more than the number of people at that time.

Timeline of The Second Wave
Africa

- 24 August: H.M.S. Mantua arrived in Sierra Leone with 200 sick sailors (none died). On 27 August, 500 of the 600 employees of the Sierra Leone Coal Company caught the flu and passed it on to their families.
- In the following week, 75% of the British crew of the H.M.S. in Africa contracted the flu. Of those 580 or so, 51 died.
- In early September 1918, a Royal Navy minesweeper, the H.M.S. Chepstow, carrying troops from New Zealand, reported 38 deaths from a stopover in Sierra Leone. Tahiti, which had military ports, reported 68 deaths within two days of the minesweeper's passage.

- At the end of September, 1,072 people in Sierra Leone (approximately 3% of the population) had died of the Flu.

France

- Brest in France was the main landing port for the American Expeditionary Force (AEF). By August 1918, there were approximately 17,000 Americans in Brest, and the nearby AEF camp housed another 45,000 troops.
- In the last days of August, many French troops, infected with the flu, arrived in Brest for training.
- The first cases of deadly flu appeared around August 22nd. On September 15, 1,350 patients were hospitalized; 370 of them died.

United States

- The first reports came out on September 8 from Camp Devens, 30 miles west of Boston.

- The camp was built for 36,000 soldiers, but at that time it was overcrowded with 45,000 men.
- On September 8, ninety flu patients attended the camp clinic. In the days that followed, the number of people hospitalized grew exponentially.
- On September 29, the clinic, built to treat 1,200 patients, had to include another 6,000 beds for those infected, row after row.
- By mid-August, more than 14,000 soldiers at Camp Devens had fallen ill; 750 had died.
- Troop movements soon spread the disease to other camps in New Jersey (Fort Dix), Kansas (Camp Funston), New York (Camp Upton), California and Georgia.
- Two soldiers arrived at Dodge Camp in Iowa on September 12; six weeks later, 12,000 men were infected; the infirmary built for 2,000 people had 8,000 patients.
- In 1918, the Philadelphia Naval Base was the largest in the United States, with 45,000 sailors.

- On September 7, 300 sailors arrived from Boston.
- Two weeks later, more than 900 sailors were sick.
- Philadelphia held a Liberty Loan campaign parade on September 28.
- 3,000 soldiers and sailors marched through streets full of more than 100,000 spectators.
- Two days later, more than 100 people died of the Flu every day.

THE THIRD WAVE

The third and last wave began in early 1919, persisted all spring and caused even more cases of illness and death. The flu would once again shake the world, although this time its mortality was generally lower than in the previous phase of infection. One of the scientists' suspicions is that the population had already built up immunity so that the strength of the virus was lower. In countries such as Japan, for example, the incidence of influenza would extend to 1920. When it was over, eight million people had already died in Spain.

While dangerous, this wave was not as deadly as the second one. The influenza pandemic finally subsided in the summer of 1919, after families and communities were wiped out and had to move on. Scientists now know that this pandemic was caused by the H1N1 virus, which continued as a seasonal virus around the world for the next 38 years.

HOW DID IT END?

The pandemic ended naturally, after about two years or so of impact. It wasn't until the 1930s that attempts were made to develop vaccines. At the time, not enough was known to develop vaccines or medicines for "new" diseases so immediately.

The underdeveloped and basic medical methods of the time did little to alleviate or slow the spread of the virus, as doctors relied on ineffective home techniques such as hot liquor or even tobacco smoke to kill the virus. In addition, at that time there was no social security and not all people had access to health care.

In some countries, adequate security measures were not taken or social events such as funerals or employers' festivities were prevented, although many public workers such as doctors or police officers were required to wear masks.

The Spanish Flu saw its end on the path of immunization, which managed to isolate it, until its extinction. There were three waves of great impact of the disease, in which a great part of the people was infected and helped the virus to go under siege. After those waves, the population was sufficiently immunized to hinder the expansion and permanence of the pandemic. The reason for the extinction of the pandemic is "herd immunity". Immunity to a virus is created by people who have been infected and have recovered, thus causing their bodies to create antibodies that are able to "fight" that specific alteration of the virus.

This immunity can be genetically transmitted from mother to child, provided that the mother was infected during pregnancy. So, after two years of infection, the virus stops spreading because there are no healthy individuals left without antibodies to infect.

LACK OF SOCIAL ESTRANGEMENT

What is true?

More people died in the 1918 flu pandemic than in the entire World War I, and most people died in the deadly second wave of the flu outbreak. In general, in places where social distance rules were not observed, there were more cases of influenza.

It's Wrong

However, the second wave of the influenza outbreak started before World War I. It was largely driven by malaise soldiers traveling to hospitals, not those who ignore the rules of social distance.

There were three waves during this pandemic, which started in the spring of 1918 and decreased in the summer of 1919, the deadliest being the second wave that peaked in the fall of 1918.

The conclusion has not been made on the percentage of deaths during the second deadly wave. However, we can say that in October 1918 alone, the United States saw almost 200,000 deaths from the pandemic. The United States lost around 115,000 soldiers during World War I.

While most deaths occurred during the second wave, these deaths cannot be attributed solely to the lack of social distance after the war. In fact, in a timeline of the Centers for Disease Control and Prevention (CDC) 1918 pandemic, it is observed that the second wave started in September 1918, approximately two months before Germany officially surrendered on November 11 and World War I will end.

The second wave of the 1918 pandemic was largely fueled by soldiers who traveled to countries in Europe, the United States, and Africa, although military parades and lack of social distance at the end of the war did not trigger the second wave of the 1918 pandemic, they did exacerbate the problem. Like today, many cities in the United States closed schools, businesses, and other public places during the 1918 pandemic. These actions were largely successful in slowing the spread of the disease.

There are also several historical examples of cities that ignored these rules only to see an increase in influenza cases. For example, Philadelphia organized a parade of 200,000 soldiers, days after they saw their first fatal case of "Spanish flu" in September 1918. St. Louis was also supposed to hold a parade at this time, but they cancelled the event due to the pandemic. No wonder Philadelphia ended up with a death rate more than double that of St. Louis.

In summary, the 1918 pandemic killed about 40 million people; more than double the death toll of World War I. While ignoring social distance rules did increase in flu cases, Armistice Day parades commemorating the end of World War I did not cause the second deadly wave as it was already underway towards the end of the World War I.

THE 1920's-1950's

In the years following the outbreak, the H1N1 virus was circulating, although it did not re-emerge to cause illness and death on a similar scale. In the decades before the re-emergence of another pandemic disease, global and public health would progress by leaps and bounds. Regarding the Spanish Flu pandemic, three areas of progress should be highlighted: the isolation and identification of viruses, the development of vaccines and the advancement of global health diplomacy.

Richard Shope was the first to isolate the influenza virus in the laboratory in 1931 and extract it from infected pigs. Shortly thereafter, Smith, Andrewes, and Laidlaw isolated the virus in humans and challenged the widespread belief that influenza was a bacterial infection. This was a major breakthrough for diagnostic, monitoring and vaccine development efforts.

The first vaccine against the influenza virus was developed in parallel by several researchers in the late 1930s and early 1940s. Jonas Salk and Thomas Francis did a great job even though during this period, vaccines were not as safe as modern ones. Impurities sometimes caused symptoms such as fever, pain and fatigue.

Meanwhile, poor monitoring capabilities made it difficult to properly match the vaccine to the circulating strain of influenza. For example, an epidemic flared up in 1947 when antigenic drift led to changes in the haemagglutinin antigen, so the vaccine offered no protection against it. Fortunately, it was not very serious, and it did not become a pandemic.

The discovery and isolation of the virus would dramatically change the way societies would respond radically to the prevention and control of an epidemic. Meanwhile, the development of penicillin in 1929 would provide health planners with an essential tool for treating secondary bacterial pneumonia, the leading cause of death during influenza pandemics.

In addition, pressure ventilators were developed in the 1940s for use in intensive care units; this would also improve health outcomes in complicated cases. These claims have helped prevent a new pandemic with a mortality rate comparable to that of the Spanish flu.

During the pandemic of 1918, there was little significant coordination between jurisdictions; there were several reasons for this. Significant international cooperation in the fight against infectious diseases was still premature. In 1851, a series of international health conferences began to bring countries together to address the control of infectious diseases; however, the first treaties to emerge from these conferences, focusing on sanitation, proved to be of limited use during an influenza pandemic. Meanwhile, international organizations with mandates to coordinate and report on the response to infectious diseases would have been inadequate.

International organizations such as the Pan American Sanitary Bureau (later to become the Pan American Health Organization) and the International Bureau of Public Health in Paris, France, were founded in the early 1900s, but were not of the size, rank or experience to contribute effectively to the Spanish Influenza response. Meanwhile, the League of Nations, possibly the world's first political system, was founded in 1919. A health organization was established in 1923 (replaced by the World Health Organization in 1948).

These international bodies would play an important role in subsequent pandemics. In addition, many national health institutions did not exist, and provincial health departments were small. In Canada, largely because of the disorganized response to the Spanish flu, legislation was established in March 1919 to create a federal department of health. In the United States, the Center for Communicable Diseases (now the Centers for Disease Control and Prevention) was formed.

As a result, states have planned and implemented very different control strategies, often with little information, based on the experience and best practices of other states. In the absence of these national and international coordinating bodies, lack of communication and reporting across jurisdictions hindered more effective responses. The scope and responsibilities of local, state, provincial and federal health departments have expanded. In the inter-pandemic period between 1918 and 1957, the world experienced tremendous growth in population, trade and travel. In 1918, the world population was about 1.8 billion; by 1957, that number had increased to 2.8 billion. Meanwhile, international travel for both business and leisure travelers has steadily increased over the years. With the advent of commercial air travel in the 1950s, the number of international travelers increased even faster.

Although the globalization of trade came to a halt between 1914 and 1945, limited by World War I, the Great Depression, and World War II, it would re-emerge again in the 1950s and the so-called "second era of globalization" (the explosion of trade, capital, and migration during the industrial revolution). The beginning of this second era dates back to the founding of the United Nations between 1944 and 1947 and three multilateral economic institutions known collectively as the Bretton Woods system: The World Bank, the International Monetary Fund and the General Agreement on fees and trade.

These organizations paved the way for unprecedented cooperation and liberalization of international trade, which would encourage the formation of multinational institutions and the international movement of goods, services and information on a completely different scale than before World War I.

Although three decades of advances in medical science, public health practice and international policy cooperation improved influenza pandemic preparedness, population growth and the globalization of trade and travel risked increasing the spread of disease. This contributed to the emergence of three global influenza pandemics, albeit mild, in this period of time:

- 1957-1958: The Asian flu, caused by the H2N2 virus, killed two million people.
- 1962: The 1962 Tanganyika (now Tanzania) Laughing Epidemic, approximately 1,000 people were affected.
- 1968-1969: The Hong Kong flu (influenza A subtype H3N2) claims one million victims.

POST-TRAUMATIC COMPLICATIONS

The excess deaths from all causes during the highly virulent second period from October to December 1918 (8.6 deaths per 1,000) was twelve times greater than the corresponding death rate during the first Flu attack from July to September 1918 (0.7 deaths per 1,000). Mortality during the third Flu attack was relatively low.

The Spanish Flu was very serious due to bacterial complications, mainly pneumonia, but also meningitis, bronchitis, and acute diarrhea. More than 2 percent of those infected with the disease globally died with an unusually high incidence of influenza during the summer wave of 1918 for young people aged 10 to 39, especially men, and a rapidly decreasing incidence of age for those over 40.

The age-specific incidence curve for the fall wave was similar to that for the summer wave. Those most affected during the first wave appear to be least affected during the second wave in 1918, probably due to acquire relative immunity. Therefore, the crossover in gender difference in incidence at the age of 10-39 years is also clear.

Age-specific mortality from influenza and pneumonia, especially excessive mortality from the Spanish Flu, have received much research attention. Despite recent and extensive efforts in molecular and paleomicrobiological research, these problems remain a mystery. Those born around 1900, identified by Gomez de Leon (1991) as high mortality cohorts, a cohort in the field of medicine is a group that is part of a clinical trial or study observed over a period of time and in this case were represented among those with the highest incidence of influenza.

However, cohorts born between 1899 (19 years in 1918) and 1904 (14 years in 1918) had relatively low mortality compared to cohorts born in 1880 (39 years in 1918).

Thus, the disease marked a large proportion of the cohorts born in 1899-09, but only a small proportion died immediately. In other words, those who were adolescents in 1918 and 1919 may have experienced significant debilitating effects on morbidity and small selection effects on mortality from Spanish flu. The interaction of viral mechanisms in the immune system is believed to have left profound chemical imprints on the health of patients. Survivors were reported to have experienced sleepiness, depression, mental distraction, low blood pressure, dizziness during work and daily life, weeks, months, or even years after suffering from the disease. It is likely that the number of people who suffered some pathology or mental condition after the flu is much higher than the estimate shows, since it is feasible that people with mild or temporary post-flu hypochondria have not seen a psychiatrist.

Hepatitis, hearing disorders, deafness, blindness and baldness (especially in girls) are other side effects that have been associated with the Spanish flu. One-third of flu survivors have also been reported to have heart problems, pulmonary tuberculosis, and kidney disease later in life (Collier 1974).

Those who had one or more complications during the illness directly in 1918-19 would succumb in greater numbers and those who maintained some symptoms or illness related to the flu after recovery, experienced higher mortality than individuals of the same age who had no contact with the virus.

There are at least three examples from the literature that support this view: First, Wasserman (1992) found that unnecessary deaths from influenza from 1918-20 were significantly and positively associated with suicide in the United States, regardless of factors such as the alcohol consumption and the number of victims during the World War I. The proposed explanations were a decrease in social inclusion (closure of schools, churches, theaters, the prohibition of large public gatherings, etc.) and the fear caused by the pandemic (the infected could die in three days).

Various suicides may also have occurred after 1920, either because of the psychological health problems of some survivors mentioned above (direct effect) or the unbearable loss of a spouse, children, or close relatives (indirect effect).

The second example of increased mortality in survivors may be a side effect of the Spanish Flu, is the mortality associated with encephalitis lethargica. Encephalitis lethargica is a rare form of encephalitis that led to an epidemic between 1917 and 1928 with millions of deaths worldwide. Those who survived were left in a state of semi-consciousness from which some emerged in the late 1960s because of treatment with the drug L-DOPA. The disease was first described by neurologist Constantin von Economo (1876-1931) in 1917. The latent pandemic left hundreds of survivors in a rare rigid paralysis with similarities to advanced Parkinson's disease. These patients, who could only communicate or move occasionally, were almost all paralyzed for life. Ravenholt and Foege (1982) largely established the link between the Spanish Flu and the possibility of contracting the encephalitis lethargica virus.

The hypothesis of the causal relationship is based on two observations, the first being that the pandemics seemed to share an etiology. The fact that the incidence of Spanish Flu and encephalitis lethargica was higher among adolescents and young adults (10-30 years), the incidence in both was higher in men than in women, supports this thesis. The second observation is that the epidemic followed the Spanish Flu pandemic in time and space.

Reports of encephalitis lethargica were found in several European countries three years before the Spanish Flu broke out into pandemic dimensions in 1918. However, recent archival and genetic research now points to a less deadly history of the virus in the first cases around 1915. This further supports the view that the encephalitis lethargica pandemic was causally related to the Spanish Flu. It is estimated worldwide that in the period 1919-1928, more than one million were infected and half a million died from the epidemic of the disease described by neurologist Constantin von Economo.

The third example of relatively high mortality after surviving the 1918 influenza pandemic is potentially associated with coronary heart disease.

Using cross-sectional data, they found that the Spanish Flu is a good predictor of the increase (1920-67) and decrease (1968-85) of coronary heart disease mortality in the United States. The analysis found that cohorts born around 1900, who had the highest exposure and mortality from the flu, also had the highest mortality from coronary heart disease later in life. Subsequently, the earlier and later cohorts had lower mortality from heart disease. Some theories suggest that the stress caused by the pandemic on mothers may have affected fetal development. Scientists found that babies born during the epidemic were more likely to develop conditions such as heart disease, compared to children born before or after the outbreak. The higher incidence of the 1918-19 Spanish flu among men than among women was also used to explain why men after the 1920s always had higher mortality from coronary heart disease than women. However, traditional risk factors such as smoking, unhealthy diet and reduced physical activity have been used to explain cyclical death.

Another clue to the genetic impact of the pandemic was found in an analysis of soldier recruitment data for the U.S. Army, which said that new recruits born in 1919 were "1mm" shorter on average than their peers.

THE ECONOMIC EFFECTS

The 1918 Flu epidemic is an important episode to study, not only because of its large size, but also because economists know little about how major demographic and occupational shocks affect economic growth, economic theory provides ambiguous predictions about the relationship. between negative demographic shocks and economic growth and the other great historical pandemics that do not provide convincing evidence of the import. The importance of understanding the relationship is further underlined by the massive loss of life due to AIDS in many developing countries; partly due to lack of evidence, the impact of the AIDS epidemic on economic decrease in these regions remains an unsolved problem. Although we highlight below the differences between the influenza epidemic and the AIDS epidemic, both are linked by the almost incomprehensible magnitude of the deaths recorded in both crises.

Post-epidemic economic decrease in the United States where we observe that it is negatively correlated, even taking into account differences in population density, urbanization, per capita income levels, climate, geography, and the sectoral composition of the production and the accumulation of human capital.

Our results suggest that one death per thousand resulted in an average annual decrease rate of real income per capita in the next decade of at least 0.15 percent per year. Newspapers in the cities of the Eighth Federal Reserve District of Little Rock and Memphis printed in the fall of 1918 were examined for information on the effects of the Flu pandemic in these cities. The merger of information from these cities can provide a relatively good picture of the overall effects of the pandemic. These general effects in 1918 can be used to extrapolate the possible economic effects of a modern pandemic.

Summary of economic research

A research paper, analyzes about the direct (short-term) effect of Flu mortality on production wages in cities and states of the United States for the period 1914-1919. The document's hypothesis is that Flu deaths directly affected industry wages during and immediately after the 1918 Flu.

The hypothesis is based on a simple economic model of the labor market: a decrease in the supply of factory workers due to deaths from influenza would initially have led to a reduction in the supply of labor in the processing industry, reducing the marginal product of labor and would increase capital per employee and thus increase real wages.

In the short term, labor immobility between cities and states has probably prevented equalization of wages in the states, and it is unlikely that relatively more expensive labor for capital has been replaced. Empirical results support the hypothesis: cities and states with the highest influenza death rate experienced the most significant increase in wages in the industry in the period from 1914 to 1919. Another study examined the state's revenue growth during the decade following the Flu pandemic using a similar methodology. In their unpublished manuscript, the authors state that states that experienced a higher death rate from influenza per capita would have experienced higher per capita income after the pandemic.

In essence, states with higher influenza death rates would have had a greater capital increase and, therefore, output per employee and higher post-pandemic incomes. Using statewide personal income estimates for 1919-1921 and 1930, the authors find a positive and statistically significant relationship between Flu mortality across the state and subsequent growth in per capita income. A recent article explored the long-term effect of the 1918 Flu.

The author wonders if exposure to influenza in the womb had adverse economic consequences for the elderly. The study came after the author examined evidence suggesting that pregnant women exposed to the Flu in 1918 had children who had larger medical problems later in life, such as schizophrenia, diabetes, and stroke. The author hypothesizes that promoting a person's health is positively related to their human capital and productivity and, therefore, wages and income. Using data from the 1960-1980 decennial censuses, the author discovered that during the 1918 pandemic, cohorts in utero had reduced levels of education, disability, and income. Specifically: "women show large and discontinuous reductions in educational level during pregnancy in the midst of the pandemic. Children of infected mothers were up to 15 percent less likely to graduate from high school. The men's wages were 5-9 percent lower due to the infection".

Overview

Most of the evidence indicates that the economic effects of the 1918 influenza pandemic were short-lived. Many companies, especially those in the service and entertainment sector, experienced double-digit earnings. Other companies specializing in health care products experienced an increase in revenue. Some academic research suggests that the 1918 Flu pandemic caused a labor shortage that resulted in workers temporarily increasing wages (at least temporarily). However, there can be no reasonable argument that this benefit outweighs the cost of loss: massive lives and economic activity in general. Research suggests that the 1918 Flu for people in the womb during the pandemic caused a reduction in human capital, affecting the economic activity that took place decades after the pandemic.

THE SOCIAL IMPACT IN AFRICA

The only control of the inexorable growth of the African population during the 20th century was incidentally caused by the influenza pandemic. Given the large size of the event, it is not surprising that its effects were felt in more than just population statistics. The epidemic triggered the "renewed" sanitation syndrome of white residents who feared they would be infected if the infection spread through black neighborhoods, further reinforcing the legally imposed call for racial segregation.

In outlining the development of segregationist legislation and the Urban Native Areas Act, the great South African historian Cornelis de Kiewiet noted that "the influenza epidemic revealed the way in which diseases were easily cultivated in small congested huts in the poorest and most unsanitary neighborhoods.

Similarly, Howard Phillips, who wrote extensively about the impact of the flu in South Africa, described how the threat of the disease was used to enforce racist law. The pandemic directly affected the survivors; "Being sad and suffering with no one to help them.

Describing the events in Bechuanaland, John Spears noted that epidemics are "the greatest challenges to human society because they divide and alienate as well as kill; there is no heroic battle against the fear of an unknown and invisible attacker. When fear forces friends and even family members to abandon each other, to escape the infectious breath of their loved ones, society can easily break apart".

In a society with a strong religious and superstitious culture in the world where survivors were trying to make sense of their existence, many came to the same conclusions as the prophet Nontetha Nkwenkwe, a middle-aged Xhosa woman who after surviving the deadly virus reported that a series of hallucinations during her convalescence revealed to her that the flu had been a punishment from God. Consequently, she embarked on a mission to transform her society. He applied numerous prohibitions and rules to his followers.

In a parallel movement, in 1919, the ancient Israelites gathered in the holy village of Ntabelanga, 200 kilometers north of Nontetha, to await the end of the world. In May 1921, police killed nearly 200 Israelis near Queenstown in a clash over attempts to drive out the settlers.

COULD A 1918 PANDEMIC REAPPEAR?

If so, what can we do about it?

In its course of disease and pathological characteristics, the 1918 pandemic was different, but not in kind, from previous and subsequent pandemics. Despite the extraordinary number of deaths worldwide, the majority of influenza cases in 1918 (in higher percentage in industrialized countries) were mild and essentially indistinguishable from influenza cases today.

In addition, laboratory experiments with recombinant influenza viruses containing genes from the 1918 virus suggest that similar viruses would be as sensitive as other typical strains of the virus to the Food and Drug Administration-approved influenza drugs rimantadine and oseltamivir.

However, some characteristics of the 1918 pandemic seem unique: in particular, death rates were 5 to 20 times higher than expected. Clinically and pathologically, these high mortality rates appear to be due to several factors, including a greater number of severe and complicated respiratory infections than the involvement of organ systems outside the normal range of the influenza virus. Furthermore, the deaths were concentrated in an unusually young age group.

Finally, in 1918, three separate recurrences of influenza followed one another at an unusual rate, resulting in three explosive pandemic waves in one year. Each of these unique traits may reflect genetic traits of the 1918 virus, but to understand them, host and environmental factors must also be explored. Until we can determine which of these factors resulted in the observed death patterns and learn more about the pandemic, predictions are just speculation.

We can only deduce that, should it occur, conditions similar to those of 1918 are impossible, but the effects on a globalized planet can be equally devastating. Like the 1918 virus, H5N1 is a bird virus, although it is distantly related, the evolutionary path that led to the emergence of a pandemic in 1918 is completely unknown, but it appears to be different in many ways from the situation with H5N1.

It is clear that the periods between the emergence of emerging diseases are becoming more common and there are no signs that this scenario will change in the future. What this fact teaches is that countries must be willing to effectively discover their arrival, have the capacity to establish what it is about and isolate the strain in order to develop vaccines, provide a timely medical and healthcare response and then, identify exactly what has produced it, achieve international unity of response, since it affects us all, epidemics know no limits, thoughts or social class.

In short, no one is prepared for such a context, and it is very possible that at another time we will be faced with another virus, whether respiratory or otherwise, since these mutate assiduously and every so often a more powerful variant is generated, for which we do not possess any kind of immunity.

In the face of future pandemics, not only will it be important for us to assume an orderly plan of response (conclusion protocols, distribution of medical resources and observance of quarantines), but we will also have to take into account grouped responses to the place that human beings and their well-being occupy in our societies. Accordingly, responses will be especially designed to deal with the social and economic damage that such contexts would entail.

PREPARING FOR THE NEXT PANDEMIC

Since the 1918 pandemic, great progress has been made in the world in understanding and dealing with influenza, but the viruses continue to pose an imminent threat to public health. An extensive reservoir of viruses circulating among animals, primarily birds, shows a strong danger that another influenza pandemic may emerge. For more than 60 years, the Centers for Disease Control and Prevention has worked to address the imminence of influenza and prepare for the next pandemic.

Viruses with pandemic potential are currently being discovered through the World Health Organization's 114-state global influenza surveillance and response method. The Influenza Division of the Centers for Disease

Control and Prevention is one of six participating centers worldwide that help monitor and track the movement of influenza and process candidate viruses for use in vaccine development. The Centers for Disease Control and Prevention also works with public health partners to monitor and track human infections with influenza viruses that come from animals, conducts ongoing laboratory studies on influenza viruses that disturb both humans and animals in order to understand the particularities of these viruses.

Seasonal influenza vaccines used to prevent infection are produced annually, and pre-pandemic influenza vaccines are also created and stored by the U.S. federal government for use during a pandemic event. Antiviral drugs that are used to treat seasonal influenza disease are one possible tool to combat a possible pandemic flu. Another major advance that has been made since the 1918 pandemic is the addition of antibiotics to treat secondary bacterial infections such as pneumonia. Some of the various medical equipment that has been developed since 1918 to help combat pandemics are respirators and intensive care units, along with personal protective equipment such as gloves, gowns and masks, which are now widely used to protect health workers from infection.

Countries around the world are also working to lessen the impact of future pandemics by supporting research that can improve the study of community containment and distancing measures (e.g., temporarily closing schools, postponing or canceling large public events, and establishing protocols for physical distance between people). These non-pharmaceutical mediations continue to be an integral component of efforts to control dissemination and, in the absence of the vaccine, would be the first line of defense.

There is still much to be done to be ready for the next influenza pandemic, there is a need for vaccines and treatment drugs that are more prodigiously effective, that can be produced quickly and less expensively, and there is also a substantial need for improved care and attention to influenza viruses in animals.

IMPACT ON MENTAL HEALTH

Epidemics are health emergencies that threaten human life and cause many sick and dead. Local resources are generally overloaded, and the security and normal functioning of the community is threatened. Therefore, external help is urgently needed. However, as with other catastrophic events, epidemics are also real human tragedies, so the sadness and psychological consequences must also be addressed.

In terms of mental health, a major epidemic involves a psychosocial disorder that may exceed the capacity of the affected population to handle the situation. It can even be said that the entire population experiences stress and anxiety to some degree. Therefore, it is estimated that the incidence of mental disorders is increasing (between a third and a half of the exposed population may show some psychopathological manifestation depending on the magnitude of the event and the degree of vulnerability). However, it should be noted that not all psychological and social problems that arise as illnesses can be described; most are normal reactions to an abnormal situation.

The effects on mental health tend to be strongest in populations living in precarious conditions, with limited resources and without access to social and health services.

Psychological Disorders in Survivors

On an individual level, many people may experience a crisis defined as a situation caused by an external life event that exceeds a person's emotional responsiveness. In essence, that person's coping skills are inadequate, and a psychological imbalance or lack of adjustment occurs.

Certain feelings and reactions often occur in highly emotionally significant situations, such as suffering a serious illness and / or the death of a loved one. In addition, the memory of what happened will be part of the victims' lives and will never be erased from their memories.

Although some psychological manifestations are the transient and understandable response to life through traumatic experiences, they can also be indicators that the person is developing a pathological condition. The evaluation must be carried out in the context of the facts to determine if these manifestations are "normal or expected" or, on the contrary if they are psychopathological manifestations that require professional assistance.

Some criteria for determining whether emotional expression becomes a symptom of something else include:
- Long-term suffering
- Intense suffering
- Associated complications (suicidal behavior)
- Significant impact on an individual's routine and social functioning.

The most common immediate psychological disorders in survivors are depression and acute transient stress reactions. The risk of these outages increases depending on the circumstances surrounding the losses and other vulnerability factors. In emergencies, an increase in violent behavior and excessive alcohol consumption has also been occasionally observed.

Some of the reported delayed effects are pathological sadness, depression, alimentation disorders, manifestations of post-traumatic stress, abuse of alcohol or other addictive substances, and psychosomatic disorders. Long-term suffering patterns also manifest as sadness, generalized anxiety, and physical anxiety, symptoms that often become severe and long-lasting.

Adjustment disorders are characterized by a state of subjective discomfort, emotional changes that affect social life, and difficulty accepting the changes caused by the loss.

Post-traumatic stress (or some of its symptoms) appears later or is a type of delayed disorder caused by exceptionally threatening or catastrophic events; Experiencing a major epidemic, especially for those who have suffered heavy losses, can cause symptoms of post-traumatic stress.

Mourning

Anguish, suffering, and grief are expected after the death of one or more loved ones. The period of mourning is when the person assimilates what happened, understands it, overcomes it, and rebuilds his life. This is a normal process and should not be rushed. Nor should you try to eliminate it or consider it a disease.

All societies have rites, rules, and ways of expressing their pain based on their different concepts of life and death. Performing the rituals established by the collective culture is an integral part of the recovery process for survivors.

Sadness is experienced as a mixture of grief, distrust, fear and anger. At the most critical

point, it reaches the extremes of intense emotional pain and despair.. At the most critical point, it reaches the extremes of intense emotional pain and despair. Then comes relief gradually, and the process ends with expressions of renewed confidence and hope. The grieving process involves:
• Free yourself or leave the relationship with the deceased
• Adapt to the world in different circumstances
• Make efforts to build new relationships

Coping with loss is closely related to the following factors:
• The personality and survival mechanisms
• The relationship with the deceased person
• Circumstances in which death occurred
• Social support network (family, friends, and community)

The most common psychological manifestations of grief are very vivid and repeated memories of the deceased and what happened, nervousness, anxiety, sadness, crying, desire to die, sleep and eating disorders, memory and concentration problems, fatigue, apathy, and Difficulty resuming normal activities, lack of motivation, and difficulty returning to a normal activity level, the tendency to isolation, mixed feelings or emotions (such as blaming yourself, blaming others, frustration, helplessness, anger, feeling overwhelmed, etc.), neglect of personal appearance and hygiene and various non-specific physical manifestations (such as dizziness, nausea, headache, chest pain, tremors, respiratory problems, palpitations, and dry mouth).

In a major catastrophe, grief means dealing with many other losses and involves a broader and more community-oriented feeling. It involves interrupting a life plan with a family dimension and a social, economic, and political dimension.

Complex grief is a grief that does not proceed "naturally" and becomes pathological. It usually leads to a major depressive disorder characterized by deep sadness, loss of interest, and the ability to enjoy, decreased activity levels, and extreme fatigue. There are other symptoms, such as decreased attention and concentration, loss of confidence, feelings of inferiority, guilt, and a bleak vision of the future, thinking or trying to commit suicide, sleep disorders, and loss of appetite.

Many circumstances can hinder the grieving process, but personal vulnerability and the extent of the loss can be listed. Complex grief often leads to the onset of psychiatric disorders that require more specialized interventions. In massive epidemics and fatal situations, several authors have described the fears and feelings of survivors:

- Sadness and suffering for the loss of family and friends, which sometimes coincides with material losses. There are also more subtle and occasionally intangible losses, such as loss of faith in God, loss of the meaning of life, etc.
- Practical fears: playing new roles imposed by the disappearance of a family member (for example, the widow who becomes the head of the household or the widower who has to take care of the children)
- Recurring fears that something may happen again or that death will happen to other family or community members.
- Personal fear of death: fear of the unknown or fear of facing God.

- Feelings of loneliness and desolation: It is common for survivors to feel that their family and friends have left them at a difficult time.
- Fear of being forgotten.
- Anger towards the deceased that is taken from close family or friends.
- Some degree of guilt over someone's death; sometimes what happens after the death of a loved one increases this guilt.
- Shame after the death of a loved one due to circumstances surrounding that person's death (their behavior, humiliation, etc.); or ashamed of the circumstances in which a family is left after a disaster.

Care of Mental Health

Experience has shown that mental health plans should not be limited to extending and improving the specialized services offered directly to those affected; the perspective should shift to a much broader area of expertise.

For example, emphasis can be placed on the relationship between mental health services and a wide range of activities, such as:
- Humanitarian and social assistance.
- Guidance for the population and risk groups.
- Mass communication.

It is also recognized that after major disasters, long-term care is needed for survivors' mental health problems. At the same time, they are tasked with rebuilding their lives. This raises the need to formulate psychosocial recovery plans in the medium and long term.

In terms of care, three periods can be distinguished (before, during, and after the epidemic), along with four groups of people:
- The sick
- Those that had the disease and survived

- Those that are not ill can get sick and have suffered significant losses (death or illness among family, friends or neighbors)
- Members of the emergency response team.

Psychological and Social Care

Initially, crisis intervention techniques will have to be used for people who are not sick but who experience significant psychological reactions. Health and humanitarian workers should be trained in basic emotional first aid techniques. It is especially important to have mental health services with crisis intervention in the main health centers where patients are cared for; creating an entity that provides care for family members and companions.

The following are recommendations for survivors and those who have suffered heavy losses:

- Treat them as active survivors and not as passive victims.
- Do not seek medical attention and do not necessarily treat people as psychiatric patients.
- Help them and show concerns about their health and physical safety.
- Make sure basic needs are met
- Provide emotional support and a sense of connection with other people.
- Guarantee privacy and confidentiality in communication.
- Help them tell their story and express their feelings.
- Develop a responsible, careful, and patient way of listening among those who provide psychological help; members of the response team should research their ideas and concerns about death and not impose it on those who help them.

- Instead of giving advice, let survivors think about what happened and how they can look to the future, therefore, the advice should cover practical issues and available help channels.
- Provide as much information as possible and listen to problems to solve them.
- Encourage a return to daily life as soon as circumstances allow.
- Avoid pressure from the press or other groups.
- Know that spiritual or religious support is often a valuable way to calm family members.

The criteria for referral to a specialist (psychologist or medical psychiatrist) are limited and specific:
- Persistent and/or worsened symptoms that have not been alleviated by the initial measures.
- Clear difficulties in family, work or social life
- Risk of complications, especially suicide.
- Coexisting problems, such as alcoholism or other addictions.

- Major depression, psychosis, and post-traumatic stress disorder are severe psychiatric conditions that require specialized care.

Medications should only be used if necessary and only if prescribed by a doctor. Long-term, random use of psychoactive drugs is not recommended. Certain medications, such as tranquilizers, have significant side effects and can lead to addiction.

The vast majority of cases can and should be treated on an outpatient basis within the family and community context. Hospitalization is generally not necessary. In everyday life, people's psychosocial recovery begins after major traumatic events. The following is recommended for surviving children:
- A flexible and non-specialized psychosocial care strategy.

- View school, community, and family as basic therapeutic forums.
- Let teachers, community workers, women's groups, and youth groups become agents who work with children.
- Strengthen the training, care, and motivation of staff who work with children.
- Group techniques that include games and recreational activities as essential tools for the psychosocial recovery of children.
- Encourage a return to normal life as soon as possible, including a return to school.
- Benefit from generally accepted traditions regarding the care and treatment of affected children.
- Basic principles of a national mental health plan in an epidemic or pandemic situation.
- The plan should not focus only on traumatic impact (epidemic disease), but should be comprehensive and encompass the individual and their context, and use positive coping

strategies with an ideological, cultural and religious focus (for those who have such beliefs).
• Goals must be realistic and objective. The main objective is prevention (reducing the risk of psychosocial harm).

The established objectives must define short, medium, and long-term actions. When conducting any activity, the responsible person and end dates must be clear.
• Psychosocial intervention must be early, fast, and efficient.
• The working methods must be fast, simple, concrete, and adaptable to ethnic and cultural characteristics.
• To begin, a rapid assessment of psychosocial needs and situations of greatest vulnerability should be made; this serves as the basis for action in the initial phase.

- Care should not be seen only in terms of clinical psychiatric care.
- The plan should create safe environments, promote community life, and support family reunification.
- Active correction should be encouraged, as reflected in the resumption of daily community activities such as work and school for children.
- Community forums should be created for mutual support, expression, exchange, understanding, and listening. The impact is social, to reevaluate, and mobilize resources.
- Affected should listen to people's demands in their own social or informal environment and not expect them to go to health services.
- Emotional support should be integrated into the daily activities of organized community groups and be part of the population's basic needs.

- Emotional support should be provided to bereaved people, with an emphasis on culturally accepted funerals and rites.
- The gender approach must be integrated.
- Associations must be established, and different social actors must participate.
- At the operational level, priority must be given to the group and the community, without prejudice to the family and the individual.
- Flexibility is necessary; the psychosocial dynamics of this type of emergency varies widely, which means that each plan must be very flexible.
- Actions must be sustainable in the medium and long term; the objective is to strengthen existing services and improve mental health.

Lines of action

1. Rapid diagnosis of the psychological and social needs of the population

2. Psychosocial care by non-specialized personnel
3. Direct specialized clinical care for people with more complex mental disorders
4. Priority care for higher-risk groups
5. Social organization, social participation, and self-sufficiency
6. Mass communication
7. Interpersonal coordination.

ORGANIZATION OF SERVICES.

Services are organized according to the resources and needs of the country or region in question.

Primary level

• Primary health care team with basic mental health training, which allows them to deal with simple psychosocial support processes (such as emotional first aid) and identify and/or refer more complex cases

• Emotional support and counseling services.

• Outpatient mental health teams (community mental health centers or others) that provide primary care support from and mobilize as needed when these services are feasible

Secondary level

- Crisis intervention units (specialized) in selected places, such as emergency centers.
- Mental health care departments in general hospitals where large numbers of influenza patients are admitted (liaison services that attend medical offices).

DEAD BODY MANAGEMENET

The presence of a large number of corpses after a pandemic arouses fear in the population due to inaccurate information about the danger they represent. There is also stress and a general feeling of sadness; the prevailing chaos and emotional climate can lead to difficult behavior. This type of situation requires appropriate psychosocial interventions for the individual and the community of leaders.

There is an inherent myth that dead bodies are dangerous and should be burned or buried quickly. Accurate information should be disseminated about the health risks to survivors who burn and handle dead bodies as a result of the pandemic.

Regardless of the capacity of the responsible authorities to manage the emergency and the epidemiological reasons that could prevent adequate treatment of the remains, measures should be taken to ensure respect for the population's customs, avoiding the use of common graves and cremation, which are generally prohibited by law and violate human rights.

The handling and disposal of corpses is a problem with serious psychological implications for the family, survivors, and other political, socio-cultural, and health problems.

About the notification of death and identification of bodies, it can be reported in a home, health center, hospital, morgue or other places. This is a critical and difficult time to handle because it can cause strong reactions.

Below are some recommendations for providing notification of death to family members:

- Before reporting, gather as much information as possible about the deceased and the event (disease progression, complications, etc.)
- Obtain information about the people living with the deceased.
- Make sure the most appropriate adult family member is the first to receive the news.
- Make a report directly and personally.
- If possible, ask two people to testify about what happened.
- Adhere to common rules of courtesy and respect.
- Do not bring the deceased's personal belongings to the interview.
- Invite family members to sit down. The people who make the report should do the same.
- Observe the environment to avoid risks and be prepared to care for children or others.

- The message must be direct and simple. Most people will realize from the environment that something terrible has happened, and their pain or fear should not be prolonged.
- Be prepared to answer questions
- Help family members notify others if the family requests it.
- Listen and attend to the immediate needs of the family, reminding them of their rights.
- Death must always be reported individually (case by case). Avoid giving such information to a group. When necessary, multiple teams or pairs should divide the work.
- People (sometimes teenagers) who face the difficult task of informing and identifying family or friends' bodies are exposed to a very traumatic situation. Those who begin to identify or receive the bodies of their loved ones can manifest this trauma through expressions of

despair, frustration, and occasional protests or disagreements with the procedures used, etc.

• Medical and mental health services should be as close as possible to where the body is identified to provide physical and emotional support to family members.

Family members generally request to see the body as soon as possible

The following is recommended:

• Mourners must decide among themselves who will see the remains.

• Do not allow family members to enter the observation area unsupervised. Competent staff should preferably provide some form of emotional support.

• Offer privacy and respect so that the family can say goodbye and even touch the body.

• Respect any type of response that family members may have at that time.

- It is almost always necessary to transport relatives to the body location.
- Provide comfortable conditions and ensure compassionate treatment where bodies are seen.

An important part of dealing with pain is the quick completion of the funeral, which should be free or accessible to low-income people. Delayed delivery of the body and uncertainty about how to pay for the funeral can cause even more suffering and suffering.

The authorities often do not attach much importance to funeral services' problems, especially in the chaos caused by an epidemic. However, it is very important for family members, and failure to do so can lead to protests and social unrest.

Psychosocial Care for Reaction Teams That Take Care of the Pandemic

A particularly vulnerable group is made up of members of the response teams working during the epidemic and the people responsible for handling the bodies. Those responsible for performing autopsies are also vulnerable; they feel overwhelmed and overloaded by the workload when mass death situations occur.

Not all employees and volunteers are suitable for these tasks; their suitability depends on a series of factors related to vulnerability and circumstances, such as age, personality, previous experiences, beliefs about death, etc. They must be well informed about the nature of the tasks they will perform, and people under 21 should not participate in or perform work with profound human impact.

Certain emergency factors increase the risk of mental disorders:
- Long-term exposure to very traumatic experiences.
- Ethical conflicts
- Simultaneous exposure to other recent trauma or stressful situations.
- History of physical or mental disorders.
- Unfavorable living conditions.
- A loose selection process for professional staff.

Members of the response team are likely to experience some difficulties in returning to their daily lives. These problems should not necessarily be considered as symptoms of illness and, above all, require family and social support.

There is no form of preliminary training or preparation for a person working with seriously injured and dead victims, which can completely rule out post-traumatic stress or other mental disorders. If severe symptoms of psychopathology appear, cases should be referred to specialized treatment.

The following are some recommendations for the care of the response team members:

- Consider the characteristics of the team and specific behavior patterns. Crew members are generally satisfied with what they have achieved and develop a spirit of altruism.
- Keeping the team active is a positive thing relieves stress and strengthens self-esteem.
- Promotion of job rotation and fixed working hours, for example, team members dealing with corpses over some time should be reassigned to other less difficult tasks.
- Encourage team members to take physical care and rest regularly.
- Those that provide emotional support must listen carefully and guarantee confidentiality

and ethical handling of personal and work situations.

- Redefine crises as growth potential.
- Involve the family in the aid and awareness processes.
- Reduce stressors and assess underlying emotional states before and during the emergency.
- Create opportunities for reflection, catharsis, and integration of experience. Recognize that someone's anger is not personal, but an expression of frustration, guilt, or concern.
- Where possible, the team involved in the emergency should participate in group advisory meetings.

Recommendations for rescuers after resuming daily life:

- Get back to your routine as soon as possible.

- Do physical and relaxation exercises.
- Get in touch with nature.
- Get plenty of rest and sleep.
- Eat balanced meals regularly.
- Don't try to reduce suffering by using drugs and alcohol.
- Find company and talk with other people.
- Participate in family and social activities.
- Observe and analyze your feelings and thoughts; reflect on what you have experienced, and its meaning in life.

At the primary level, the Primary Health Care (PHC) team must have basic mental health training so that it can handle simple psychosocial support processes. Emotional support and counseling, as well as outpatient mental health teams that support PHC, should also be anticipated.

At the secondary level, it is important to plan crisis intervention units in selected areas (such as emergencies and morgues) and for mental health care in general, hospitals where there are many influenza patients. The delayed effects (in the medium and long term) that occur in catastrophic situations should be considered when designing appropriate intervention strategies for their effective prevention and control. However, the most common institutional responses are based on individual psychiatric care and only reach a very limited number of affected people.

MASS COMMUNICATION STRATEGIES

The availability of truthful, transparent and timely information is vital for the emotional restraint of family members and the general population.

Community authorities and leaders must be willing to provide information directly to individuals or groups, but also to answer questions and be ready to find answers to these questions.

The media have a double character: on the one hand, they are for-profit companies, and, on the other hand, they have an enormous social responsibility for the public services they offer. Disaster information, such as pandemics, can be used to fuel and manipulate the public's morbid interest. However, it is necessary to insist on ethical and sensitive reports on these events; the media must make a responsible contribution to the tranquility of citizens by providing truthful and balanced information.

A common problem is the number of people who go to hospitals, health centers, morgues, and other places in search of family or friends (sick or dead). This causes congestion and disorganization problems. Solutions must be found for these situations that are adequate, humane, and respectful of these people.

The health sector must coordinate with law enforcement and humanitarian aid organizations to conquer, care for, and control crowds. In most cases, the crowd is not aggressive, but they must organize so they can get the right information. Access to health facilities should also be limited to individuals or small groups.

For these communication tasks, it is important to seek the support of neighbors and civil society organizations with extensive knowledge of the population, their customs and human talent.

It is advisable that public authorities and institutions have spokespersons specifically responsible for information management and can turn to the population for emotional restraint. It is advisable to have regular briefings and use official bulletins to avoid ambiguities.

Informing the public about the possibility of a major pandemic is not an option, but a step that must be taken without question. The reasons are clear:

• People can be prepared and can help prepare those around them (family, community, workplace, etc.).

• The community can cooperate with the official efforts of the government and other authorities.

- Once the epidemic is underway, informed people can better protect themselves and their families.

Risk communication is essential, and the basic strategy is to create an atmosphere of mutual trust between people, authorities, and communicators.

Before the epidemic breaks out, the goal of communication is to reach a midpoint where accurate information about existing risks and dangers is provided, creating an appropriate level of fear in awareness while helping to tackle the problem and prepare the population. The goal is to avoid extremes, that is, the lukewarm announcements that do not break the apathy of the population, or the alarming reports that arouse great fear and can cause panic.

Risk communication is vital from a mental health point of view. A good mass communication strategy is critical to maintaining a calm and appropriate emotional state; a well-informed population can act appropriately, protect itself better, and be less vulnerable in terms of psychosocial aspects.

CONCLUSIONS

Facing an epidemic emergency that has caused a large number of sick and dead is not only a problem for the health sector; other actors such as government agencies, NGOs, local authorities, and the community itself are involved.

The most common immediate measures to help create a climate of order and emotional calm include:

• Obtain a correct and orderly response from the authorities.

• Provide truthful and timely information; a good mass communication strategy is essential to maintain calm and an appropriate emotional state during all phases (before, during and after)

• Promote inter-institutional cooperation and community participation.

• Guarantee basic health services, including the psychosocial component. Prioritize mental health care for the most vulnerable groups, taking into account gender and age differences.

• Provide emotional first aid to the sick and their families, largely through efficient healthcare and humanitarian aid.

• Anticipate an increase in the number of people with symptoms of unresolved sadness or psychiatric disorders and provide appropriate care for them.

• Ensure the careful and ethical management of the bodies, establishing an orderly and individualized death report system.

• Avoid cremation or burial in communal graves. Support the rapid transfer of relics to family members so that the wishes and customs of the population can be respected.

• Mental health services should be organized as needed in an epidemic situation.

Depending on the culture, traumatic experiences, losses and pain necessarily take different forms of expression. The prevailing concepts of life and death and funeral rites for loved ones are important in accepting and understanding what happened.

This review examined how the understanding, experience and response to the Spanish Flu Pandemic has evolved over time. While significant progress has been made in mitigating the effects of a pandemic, largely due to advances in pharmaceutical interventions and surveillance, there is still little in the 1918 influenza pandemic.

Pandemics are inherently uncertain and require flexible policies to respond to outbreaks as they develop.

While knowledge can be gained from past experience, it is unlikely that the next event will imitate the past. Continued efforts are required to improve local, national and international surveillance, coordination and resource planning to reduce and manage future outbreaks as effectively as possible. Despite all the uncertainty that surrounds influenza pandemics, history has shown that they occur in cycles, albeit unpredictable, and the question is not when another one will occur, but whether one is ready to deal with it.